Your Guide to Getting Fit

SECOND EDITION

Your Guide to Getting Fit

Ivan Kusinitz
York College, City University of New York

Morton Fine
York College, City University of New York

Mayfield Publishing Company
Mountain View, California
London • Toronto

Library of Congress Cataloging-in-Publication Data
Kusinitz, Ivan.
    Your guide to getting fit / Ivan Kusinitz, Morton Fine. —2nd ed.
       p.   cm.
    Includes index.
    ISBN 1-55934-010-X (pbk.)
    1. Physical fitness.   I. Fine, Morton.   II. Title.
GV481.K86   1991
613.7—dc20   90-22691
                                                           CIP

Manufactured in the United States of America
10   9   8   7   6   5   4   3

Mayfield Publishing Company
1240 Villa Street
Mountain View, California

Sponsoring editor, James Bull; managing editor, Linda Toy; production editor, April Wells; copy editor, Helene Harrington; text and cover designer, Paula Goldstein; cover photographer, © 1990, David Madison; illustrator, Natalie Hill. The text was set in 10/12 Century Old Style and printed on 50# Finch Opaque by the Banta Company.

Appendix C is excerpted from *Taking Charge of Your Weight and Well-Being,* by Joyce D. Nash and Linda Ormiston, by permission of Bull Publishing Company.

Contents

2   Physical Fitness Training Principles   30

3   Cardiorespiratory Endurance   39

8 | Model Weight Loss Program   173

9   Managing Stress   194

10   Choosing a Fitness Facility   203

11   Programs for Special Needs   209

12   Common Training Questions Answered   221

13   Getting Started and Keeping Going   240

Preface

All too often textbooks advocate a lock-step approach to physical fitness. *Your Guide to Getting Fit* is different. This book supports the premise that the best physical fitness program accommodates each individual's lifestyle; we believe that this is best accomplished when the individual designs his or her own program. In our view, the student is the architect; this text provides the basic information and outlines the process, and the instructor, as fitness expert, serves as guide and advisor. In short, this book invites the college-level adult to share in the educational process of designing and implementing a personal fitness program.

APPROACH

Although the information in this book is scientifically sound, it is plainly written for students who have no grounding in physiology; its purpose is to be clear and uncomplicated. It also recognizes the diversity among students who seek fitness: needs and interests vary tremendously. This book offers students an unlimited variety of exercise options, which provides a good foundation for successful, personalized fitness programs. Faced with a student body at York College of the City University of New York whose backgrounds and needs were unusually diverse, we recognized that it was unrealistic to expect a simple theoretical base and a few traditional fitness activities to launch students into a lifelong pursuit of physical fitness. What we came up with works—it has been honed and polished over fifteen years of use by thousands of

York College students whose input and feedback have guided us. This text was also influenced by the personal exercise histories of more than one thousand readers of *Consumer Reports*. Exercisers and nonexercisers from all across the country enthusiastically described their exercise experiences in response to a brief request in *Consumer Reports* magazine. (The results of our poll appeared in *Physical Fitness for Practically Everybody,* Consumer Reports Books, 1983.) With all this diverse input, we wrote a practical text designed for today's diverse student body.

Throughout the book, we call on students to take an active part in planning and designing. In Chapters 1, 3, 4, 5, 8, and 13, students will complete worksheets ("fitness profiles") that assess their current fitness and provide the basis for moving toward a healthier lifestyle—one in which regular exercise plays a significant role. Chapter 7 offers model exercise programs, and Appendix B contains a comprehensive list of sports and activities from which students can create personalized programs. Chapters 8 and 13 provide the framework for actual program design. Here students can follow a step-by-step procedure to build a program, concluding with a personal contract consistent with practical behavior modification techniques.

ORGANIZATION

Independent action is the thrust of Chapter 1. Here readers are introduced to the meaning of physical fitness and to its components, but more importantly they assess their level of physical fitness and begin to recognize the potential of regular exercise. This sets the stage for establishing personal fitness goals that will later become the basis of the personal fitness program.

Chapter 2 introduces the training principles that are the foundation of all exercise programs. Without this information, exercisers often feel aimless as their enthusiasm flags. In nontechnical language, the chapter clearly and concisely answers questions such as: What type of exercise should I pursue? How hard should I exercise? How long? How often?

Chapters 3, 4, and 5 discuss the five components of health-related physical fitness: cardiorespiratory endurance, body composition, muscular strength, muscular endurance, and flexibility. Commonly asked questions are clearly answered.

Chapter 6 contains the basics of proper eating habits and accurate information about the important food nutrients.

Chapter 8 and Appendix B afford opportunities for readers to tinker with exercise systems and activities; this "hands-on" experience is valuable for planning a program consistent with personal goals. To help students get started, Chapter 7 contains model exercise programs that can be followed without modification. Students at any level of fitness can experiment with models in eight general categories; we present five different walking/running programs, resistance and stretching programs, and systems for exercising at home.

Appendix B concisely lists and evaluates more than 50 sports and activities. Students can analyze favorite activities to better understand their potential fitness benefits. Appendix B also contains the calorie costs of various aerobic activities.

Students whose major goal is to lose or control body fat will find a model weight control program in Chapter 8. This model is an integrated system that blends proper eating behavior and exercise as the most realistic approach to managing the problem of excessive body fat.

Chapters 9 through 12 deal with special issues and programs that have been identified by our students and by *Consumer Reports* readers. Questions related to stress management have surfaced recently in connection with physical fitness. This topic is discussed in Chapter 9, and several stress reduction techniques are presented. In Chapter 11, exercise ideas are described to meet a variety of special health concerns ranging from diabetes to pregnancy. Chapter 12, a question-and-answer chapter, places exercise in context with such specific issues as dress, weather, and common injuries.

Finally, Chapter 13 pulls it all together as readers follow the step-by-step process to get started and keep going with an individualized fitness program. This section is the heart of our York College experience; we guide students through the goal-setting and activity-selection processes toward the development of a specific program that includes a contract commitment along with start-up, maintenance, and assessment suggestions.

Although this book can be read straight through, it makes equally good sense to skim Chapter 13 after completing Chapter 1. In this way, the process will remain clear as readers use other chapters to help understand the scope of creating a personalized exercise program.

FEATURES

- *Fitness Profiles*   These twenty-five worksheets provide students with opportunities to assess, calculate, experiment, clarify, and evaluate their personal fitness behaviors.
- *Chapter Objectives*   These realistic objectives clearly set forth what can be accomplished in each chapter.
- *Model Exercise Programs*   Fourteen step-by-step exercise programs allow students to experiment with exercise systems such as weight training, interval training, and circuit training.
- *Model Weight Loss Program*   This seven-step behavior-modification approach to controlling body fat contains the ingredients essential to successfully and permanently combining proper eating habits and regular exercise in a healthy lifestyle.
- *Sports and Activities*   Fifty sports and activities are rated, based on their potential for developing each of the five components of health-related physical fitness.
- *Calorie Costs*   The calorie costs of exercise, sports, and routine activities are presented in terms of estimated calories per pound of body weight per minute. From this information students can calculate personal calorie costs.
- *Menu Planning*   A food exchange list and guidelines for planning weekly and daily menus are provided.

- *Tips for Evaluating Health Clubs*   Specific suggestions help students make in-formed decisions about clubs and spas.
- *Special Needs*   Special exercises and modifications provide students who have medically related problems with practical advice.

NEW TO THIS EDITION

This edition retains all of the special features and qualities of the original book, with the addition of new and updated information. Here are some highlights of the changes and additions:

- There is a more extensive discussion of coronary artery disease and the risk fac-tors of this widespread disease, which is the number one cause of death in the United States. The discussion focuses on those risk factors that can be influenced by changes in lifestyle.
- There is an expansion of the discussion of cholesterol and fat intake as related to heart disease. The recommendations of the National Cholesterol Education Pro-gram are presented, and the roles of tropical oils and fish oil are explained.
- Up-to-date information on exercise and metabolism has been added.
- Information on weight training safety is expanded, and exercise machine alter-natives to the free-weight exercises in the model weight training program are described.
- New home exercise equipment is evaluated, including the Nordic ski trainer, stair climber, and motorized treadmill.
- A student stress scale is provided to help identify the life events which are gener-ally classified as stressors.
- Recommended exercise heart rates are provided for pregnant women.
- Managing acute injuries via RICE (rest, ice, compression, and elevation) is explained.
- Many new explanations clarifying technical information on fitness and exercise have been inserted throughout this edition.

ANCILLARIES

We recognize that the college instructor is in the best position to decide about course content, course organization, class management, instructional materials, and teach-ing styles. It is not our place to presume otherwise. We prepared our Instructor's Manual as a kind of teaching assistant, one that can be used to support various teach-ing preferences. As instructors we have always appreciated simple, readily accessible teaching materials; this manual goes further than most instructor's guides in providing such materials.

In addition to the usual contents of many instructor's guides, this manual provides masters of each fitness profile from the text so that the instructor can duplicate them for student use and collection. Masters of laboratory worksheets are also provided to supplement the fitness profiles and to integrate the text. Here are some features of the Instructor's Manual for *Your Guide to Getting Fit:*

- *Duplication Masters* so that you can replicate the twenty-five personal fitness profiles from the text.
- *Laboratory Worksheets,* duplication masters that represent each chapter and supplement the fitness profiles.
- *Transparency Masters* of key tables, figures, and illustrations from the text to support your lecture and laboratory sessions.
- *References* that fully document the text's rigorous research.

The Instructor's Manual also contains chapter overviews, class management suggestions, tips for fitness testing, sample test questions for each chapter, schematics that tie topics to overhead transparencies, references by chapter, and organizational alternatives. This manual will help you allocate your time in ways that you consider most productive.

ACKNOWLEDGMENTS

We are indebted to the students and physical education faculty of York College of the City University of New York for the parts they played in the development of this book. We are grateful to the editors of Consumer Reports Books and to their medical advisors for their guidance and support throughout the project.

In addition, we'd like to thank the following reviewers for their many incisive comments: Jacqueline Asbury, Lynchburg College; Thomas Fahey, California State University, Chico; Maureen Henry, El Paso Community College; and Tony Zaloga, Frostburg State University.

Your Guide to Getting Fit

1

How Fit Are You?

After you've read this chapter, you will be able to:

Identify your place on the fitness continuum.

Decide whether you need medical clearance before starting an exercise program.

Assess your current physical activity patterns.

Define physical fitness and each of its five components.

Assess your current level of physical fitness in terms of the five components.

Identify your physical fitness goals and each of the fitness components involved in achieving them.

If you're unsure about physical fitness—what it is, how to achieve it, how fit you need to be, and how it relates to good health—you're not the only one. To some, physical fitness is a sacred article of faith, an eternal verity. John F. Kennedy ranked it along with mental, moral, and spiritual fitness as essential to the nation's strength. At the opposite end of the spectrum are people who think physical fitness is something for others to work at (combat soldiers, say, or professional athletes and their coaches). Some of these people eschew guilt and agree with Robert M. Hutchins, former University of Chicago president, who is supposed to have said that whenever he felt the desire to exercise, he lay down until the feeling passed.

Between the extremes, of course, are the great majority who agree that, however hard it may be to define, physical fitness is a desirable condition to be cultivated in a variety of ways and for a variety of reasons. In that large group belong most of our students and *Consumer Reports* readers. They include the following exercisers:

Amy, a college freshman who does aerobic dancing daily to keep trim

Sherman, who, having recovered from a heart attack, regularly walks or rides his bicycle to improve his cardiorespiratory endurance

Carlyle, a 21-year-old who lifts weights and plays tennis to help him feel and look better (he also believes the exercises may help him live longer)

Denise, a 35-year-old whose incentive to stick to running every day is a husband who likes her to look slim

Jim, 20, who wants to "build a powerful, muscular body"

Steve, a 41-year-old "confirmed runner" who competes against his own goals ("I win only against myself and for myself") and has "growing old with quality" in mind

Sarah, a 19-year-old varsity basketball player who stays in shape by lifting weights and practicing yoga

What physical fitness is *not,* clearly, is the same thing for everyone—a precise, readily definable entity with a single fixed standard to be applied universally.

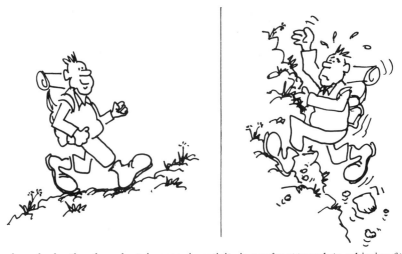

A gradual rather than sharp increase in activity is a safer approach to achieving fitness.

One useful approach to understanding physical fitness has been suggested by the President's Council on Physical Fitness and Sports. Based on the council's approach, physical fitness can be characterized as the ability to carry out daily tasks without becoming fatigued and with ample energy left to enjoy regular leisure-time pursuits and to handle an occasional unexpected emergency requiring physical exertion. The council's definition also includes the ability to last, to bear up, and to persevere under difficult circumstances.

The council describes a scale of physical fitness, ranging from "abundant life" at one extreme to "death" at the other. If you're alive, according to this view, you have at least some degree of physical fitness. Admittedly, that degree could be minimal for the severely ill or handicapped. In the highly trained athlete, of course, the degree of physical fitness would be maximal. And it could even vary in the same person at different times. Your own level of fitness is probably shaped to a great extent by *your routine—the classes you take, the needs of your job, your sports interests, the stairs you climb, or your daily rush to get to classes on time.*

THE PHYSICAL FITNESS CONTINUUM

The full spectrum of physical fitness can be envisioned as a continuum—a horizontal line on which each individual's physical fitness level is slotted in the appropriate point (see Figure 1-1). At the extreme left are those who need help to perform the routine chores of daily life. At the extreme right are healthy athletes, trained and conditioned for competition. Others are at the points along the line that reflect their lifestyle and job requirements.

If you're fit enough to perform the physical activities called for by your way of life, you might be quite content with your place on the fitness continuum. A problem could arise, however, should you take on new activities, need to get back in shape after illness, or misjudge your level of fitness. For those in good condition, a task such as shoveling snow or splitting logs can be invigorating and enjoyable. For those in poor shape, however, a vacation spent skiing may seem like a sentence to hard labor.

Take, for example, two friends who tried cross-country skiing for the first time. One was exhilarated. After a few falls, she got the hang of it and was able to negotiate an easy trail and even attempt a moderate hill. Her friend, on the other

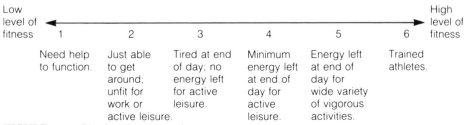

FIGURE 1-1   Physical fitness continuum.

hand, was exhausted. For him, the venture was a disaster. It began with his ski pants, last used several years before. They were so tight he had difficulty bending over to fasten his boots to his skis. Climbing a moderate hill and holding his position were difficult. His muscles seemed to "give out," and he fell repeatedly. His arms and legs ached from the unaccustomed motions of striding and reaching. He stopped repeatedly to catch his breath. After fifteen minutes, he felt his limbs grow weary with the weight of clothing and equipment; he was tempted to quit. By the end of the first half hour, he had become so frustrated that he took off his skis and returned to the lodge. Although, like his friend, he had wanted to get outdoors to enjoy the winter landscape, he ended up feeling that cross-country skiing was too much for him.

The more successful of the two cross-country skiers, with her ability to undertake a new and strenuous sport, demonstrated better-than-average fitness. She would place near 5 on the fitness continuum. Her companion would more likely place between 3 and 4. Both, in fact, are college seniors carrying heavy course loads, but the woman bikes eleven miles to and from the campus every day and plays tennis twice a week. The man drives to classes and jogs a half-mile on Sundays (if the weather is nice). With some changes in his routine, however, he could improve his level of fitness enough to enjoy cross-country skiing.

Even people with medical problems can improve their place on the fitness continuum with gradual increases in activity. Consider Rob, who is a diabetic. He has had repeated trouble controlling his blood-sugar level. Overprotected by his mother, his lifestyle was completely sedentary. This changed once he entered college. With help from the college health service and the physical education department, he began a gradual exercise program. "I started on a limited walking program and now, four months later, I am running three miles, three times a week, and riding a bike on the other days." His blood sugar is under control with less medication, and he has more than enough energy to keep up with his college work.

Like many people, you may find yourself lower on the fitness continuum than you'd like to be. If you want to improve your physical fitness by increasing your level of activity, the first step is to decide whether you need clearance from your physician. You will be able to decide for yourself once you have reviewed the guidelines that follow.

GUIDELINES FOR MEDICAL CLEARANCE

In general, if you are under 35, have no physical complaints, and have had a medical checkup within the past two years, it is probably safe for you to begin an exercise program at your current level of physical activity and gradually increase it.

Regardless of your age, consult your physician before beginning a fitness program *if:*

You are not feeling well

You have specific health concerns

You experience leg cramps with brisk walking

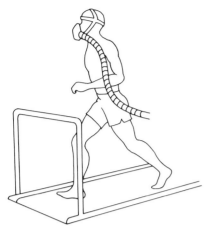

FIGURE 1-2   Cardiac stress test.

You experience shortness of breath when others don't

You are 20 percent over your desirable weight and much of the excess is body fat

You have been sedentary for a long time

You have a history of any cardiovascular disease

You are 35 or older or have a history of any of the following risk factors for coronary heart disease:

- Diabetes
- Hypertension
- High blood cholesterol levels
- A blood relative who had a heart attack before age 60
- Cigarette smoking

If you are unsure whether you have any of the risk factors, you should touch base with your physician and determine the advisability of a checkup. Your physician may require you to undergo a cardiac stress test (exercise tolerance test) before beginning a fitness program (Figure 1-2).

If you have been exercising regularly, you should be able to increase your level of activity gradually, without incurring any health problems. (Profile 1-1 can help you decide, if you have any questions.)

ESTIMATING YOUR LEVEL OF ACTIVITY

Once you've decided whether you should obtain medical clearance before making a change in your exercise program, you might find it helpful to clarify just how active you really are. We suggest that you take the series of tests described in this chapter (pp. 12–15 and pp. 18–25) to assess your physical fitness. The tests will enable you

YOUR FITNESS PROFILE 1-1
Calculating Your Activity Index

Objective: To determine your activity index on the basis of how hard, how long, and how often you exercise.

Directions: Rate the intensity, duration, and frequency of your current exercise patterns according to the criteria listed in the table. Then calculate your activity index, using the formula at the end of the table (intensity × duration × frequency = activity index). Suppose you are a skilled tennis player. Your intensity score for competitive singles would be 4; if the match lasts for an hour or more each time, your duration score would be 5; if you play regularly twice a week, your frequency score would be 2. Multiply 4 × 5 × 2 to get your activity index of 40 (moderate active). If, however, your exercise is limited to playing table tennis twice a week, your index would be 20 (2 × 5 × 2), or low active.

Rating: Your intensity _____ × your duration _____ × your frequency _____ = your activity index _____ .

Assessing your activity index: Here's how you can translate your activity index into your estimated level of activity.

If your activity index is:	Your estimated level of activity is:
Less than 15	Sedentary
15–24	Low active
25–40	Moderate active
41–60	Active
Over 60	High active

Intensity: How Hard Do You Exercise?

If your exercise results in:	*Your intensity score is:*
No change in pulse from resting level	0
Little change in pulse from resting level—as in slow walking, bowling, yoga	1
Slight increase in pulse and breathing—as in table tennis, active golf (no golf cart)	2
Moderate increase in pulse and breathing—as in leisurely bicycling, easy continuous swimming, rapid walking	3
Intermittent heavy breathing and sweating—as in tennis singles, basketball, squash	4
Sustained heavy breathing and sweating—as in jogging, cross-country skiing, rope skipping	5

Duration: How Long Do You Exercise?

If each session continues for:	*Your duration score is:*
Less than 5 minutes	0
5 to 14 minutes	1
15 to 29 minutes	2
30 to 44 minutes	3
45 to 59 minutes	4
60 minutes or more	5

Frequency: How Often Do You Exercise?

If you exercise:	*Your frequency score is:*
Less than 1 time a week	0
1 time a week	1
2 times a week	2
3 times a week	3
4 times a week	4
5 or more times a week	5

Intensity × Duration × Frequency = Activity Index

to make a relatively simple assessment of your physical fitness by evaluating your cardiorespiratory endurance, body composition, muscular strength, muscular endurance, and flexibility. Then, in Profile 1-9 you will find space to note the results of these tests as well as any comments you'd like to record. The process will help guide you in selecting the activities for your physical fitness program.

Some of the tests are strenuous and require that you be somewhat active in order to take them. Like many people, you may not be sure how to judge whether you are "somewhat" active. How does your daily run or your weekly tennis game rate? To make a simple estimate of how active you are, examine your current exercise patterns. Use Profile 1-1 to score your current exercise patterns in terms of intensity (how hard), duration (how long), and frequency (how often). Then multiply these scores to get an estimate of your level of activity.

Your activity index provides a rough estimate of your level of activity over the past three months and a very rough indication of your physical fitness. Its main purpose, at this point, is to help you decide whether it is safe to proceed to a more strenuous—and far more accurate—assessment of your physical fitness.

Regardless of your index, it's probably safe to take most of the self-assessment tests except for the 1.5-mile run-walk, which requires a higher level of activity—40 or more on the index.

The activity index can also help you decide whether you can safely increase your usual round of physical activities. If your current schedule of activities gives you an index of 41 or more (active to high active), you are probably sufficiently fit to enjoy a wide variety of vigorous activities. Increasing your exercise program would probably cause little strain. If your index is between 25 and 40 (moderate active), then you should proceed a little more slowly. If, however, your index is between 15 and 24 (low active), approach any significant increase in activity very gradually and with caution.

Indeed, if before their vacation the two novice cross-country skiers had used the activity index for even a rough assessment of their state of physical fitness, the one who experienced frustration and failure might have realized he would be too out of shape to enjoy so strenuous an outing. And if he had also taken the battery of self-assessment tests described later in this chapter, he would have found out that it was inadequacies in the five major components of health-related physical fitness that led to his failure as a cross-country skier.*

THE FIVE COMPONENTS OF FITNESS

Although differences of opinion persist as to how best to define physical fitness, most authorities have come to agree that health-related physical fitness can best be mea-

---

*Factors that are not health related that affect successful participation in a sport such as cross-country skiing include balance, agility, coordination, and speed—all having to do with motor ability, not physical fitness.

sured by performance in five components: cardiorespiratory endurance, body composition, muscular strength, muscular endurance, and flexibility (see Table 1-1).

The experiences of the cross-country skiers demonstrate how people can differ in terms of the components of physical fitness. The out-of-shape skier had difficulties with all five of them. His shortness of breath indicates lack of *cardiorespiratory endurance* (*CRE*)—the ability to perform moderately strenuous activity over an extended period of time. CRE is a measure of how well the heart and lungs supply the body's increased need for oxygen during sustained physical effort.

Sensations of heaviness and clumsiness and the feeling that clothes no longer fit properly reflect *body composition*—the relative proportion of fat to bone and muscle. A professional athlete probably has a more favorable body composition (less fat and more muscle) than a sedentary college professor, even though their height and weight may be the same.

The skier's failure to climb a moderate hill with ease and to hold his position shows lack of *muscular strength*—the ability to exert maximum force, usually in a single exertion. Lifting a heavy weight or taking a step up the side of a mountain is a measure of muscular strength.

A feeling of exhaustion and the sensation that muscles seem to "give out" relate to lack of *muscular endurance*—the ability to repeat a particular action many times or hold a particular position for an extended time. With greater endurance, it is less likely your body will feel sore or muscle-bound after exercising. If you have the muscular strength to do one sit-up yet cannot do five, it is probably muscular endurance that is the limiting factor.

Restrictions in movement are likely when there is limited *flexibility,* which is the ability to flex and extend each joint, such as the elbow or the knee, through its maximum range of motion. To proceed up even a moderate hill, a skier needs some flexibility in the hips, knees, and ankles. To manipulate a ski pole, a skier needs flexibility in the shoulders, elbows, and wrists.

The successful cross-country skier, with her ability to undertake a new and strenuous sport, demonstrates better-than-average CRE. Her body composition is relatively lean and muscular, not fat and flabby. Despite spending most of her day sitting in classes, her muscular strength and endurance are adequate, and her joints are flexible. In short, she's in pretty good condition and would rate well on all five fitness components.

TABLE 1-1   The Five Components of Physical Fitness

Physical fitness component	*Definition*
Cardiorespiratory endurance	Ability to do moderately strenuous activity over an extended period of time.
Body composition	Percentage of the body that is fat.
Muscular strength	Ability to exert maximum force in a single exertion.
Muscular endurance	Ability to repeat movements over and over or to hold a particular position for a prolonged period.
Flexibility	Ability to move a joint easily through its full range of motion.

Cardiorespiratory Endurance

The primary component of physical fitness, CRE is a measure of the ability of the heart and lungs to support moderately strenuous activity over an extended period of time.* At all levels of activity, from sleep to running, it is the cardiorespiratory system that transports oxygen from inhaled air through the bloodstream to the working muscles of the body.

Your pulse before getting out of bed in the morning might be 60 beats per minute or lower. As your day progresses with its usual round of activities, your pulse tends to fluctuate as activity levels change. The more strenuous your activity, the more oxygen you need, and the harder your cardiorespiratory system must work. In a person with high CRE, the muscles used in a CRE activity will be more effective at using oxygen than in a person with low CRE. And when CRE is high, the heart and lungs work less hard for any given activity level than when CRE is low.

If occasional vigorous activity or some relatively light daily task leaves you panting with your heart pounding for more than just a few minutes, you probably have inadequate CRE. Low CRE is most often associated with inactivity, aging, obesity, illness, and smoking.

The most accurate way to evaluate CRE is to measure the amount of oxygen actually used during strenuous exercise. This measurement can be done at the same time as a cardiac stress test, making use of a treadmill or a stationary bicycle ergometer (an apparatus used in stress testing). During exercise your breath may be directly analyzed, or, more commonly, oxygen consumption is computed from work load and heart rate measurement.

The cardiac stress test makes use of elaborate equipment, requires professional supervision and evaluation, and is costly. For many people about to begin an exercise program, such precise measurement of CRE is not necessary. By taking your pulse before and after strenuous exercise, you can make your own rough evaluation of your CRE because there is a close correlation between CRE and the heart rate response to exercise. For most people, the faster the pulse for a given intensity and duration of exercise, the less efficient the cardiorespiratory system is in delivering oxygen to the body. The slower the pulse for that amount of exercise, the higher your CRE. When CRE is high, you not only perform more efficiently but your pulse returns to a resting level more quickly after exercise.

Taking the modified step test will give you a test of CRE that you can use to begin your self-evaluation. The original Harvard Step Test, developed at the Harvard Fatigue Laboratory, has been modified somewhat in the description below. Designed for ages 10 to 69, the modified step test is based on the fact that the heart rate of someone who is physically fit increases less during exercise and returns to normal faster after exercise than does the heart rate of someone who is not physically fit. To take the modified step test, follow the directions in Profile 1-2 and then check your ratings.

---

*The terms *aerobic endurance* and *aerobic fitness* are sometimes used synonymously with CRE.

The 1.5-mile run-walk test is designed to measure your CRE by determining how much time it takes you to cover the 1.5-mile distance. It is recommended for individuals who are healthy and moderately active (a score of 40 or higher on your activity index). Originally developed by the eminent physiologist Bruno Balke, it has been used by Dr. Kenneth Cooper as part of his aerobics system.

A six- to ten-week training period is recommended for individuals who are not very active and who do not include some kind of running in their regular exercise program.

This field test has a moderate to high relationship to the cardiac stress test. It can be particularly useful to chart your progress as you move ahead with your program.

If you wish to use this test, carefully follow the directions in Profile 1-3 and determine your rating by consulting the table within it.

Body Composition

The second of the five fitness components, body composition, should not be confused with body weight. As noted earlier, a professional athlete probably has a more favorable body composition—more muscle and less fat—than an inactive college professor, even though both are the same height and weight.

Weight, nevertheless, does play some part in body composition. A standard height and weight chart, however, usually provides a considerable range of so-called ideal weights for any given height. (See chart in Appendix A.) How you assess your weight according to the chart will depend to some extent on your body build. For example, the "ideal" weight of a woman 5 feet 5 inches may be anywhere from 111 to 142 pounds, depending on her body build. The smaller her body build, the closer her weight should be to the lower end of the desirable weight range given for her height on the chart. The size of your wrist gives you a good idea of your body build. A woman 5 feet 5 inches whose wrist measures 5 inches around, for example, should be closer to 111 than to 142 pounds. You can use Profile 1-4 to help you decide whether your body build is small, medium, or large.

While the "ideal" numbers in the familiar height and weight charts have their limitations, they may be of some use in assessing body composition. (They can at least confirm evidence based on subjective findings such as the mirror test, discussed below.) A weight much higher than average for your height may suggest problems in body composition, especially if you are relatively inactive. A steady increase in weight over the years or an increase in your waist measurement are both fairly accurate indications that a disproportionate amount of the extra weight is likely to be in the form of fat, not muscle. In other words, your body fat percentage is probably high.

Because lean body tissue is denser than fat (muscle sinks, for example, while fat floats), underwater weighing is the most accurate means of assessing body composition. If the well-trained athlete and the inactive college professor were weighed under water, the athlete would weigh more because the denser muscular tissue would displace more water than the less dense fatty tissue. Underwater weighing is not

PROFILE 1-2

YOUR FITNESS PROFILE 1-2
Taking the Modified Step Test

Objective: To complete 3 minutes of stepping at 24 steps per minute. *Warning:* If you have pain under or around your knee caps, it is probably not a good idea to take a step test. The step test, or climbing up and down stairs, can result in excessive compression on the underside of the knee cap and cause pain. Check with your doctor if you are unsure of the safety of this test for someone with your knee condition.

Directions:

1. Ask someone with a stopwatch or sweep-second hand to time you.
2. At the signal to begin, step up (start with either foot) on a stair or bench that is 8 inches from ground level and then step down again. Continue stepping up and down, alternating feet, for three consecutive minutes at a rate of 24 steps per minute—about 2 steps every five seconds. (A metronome can help you maintain the rhythm.)
3. Stop at exactly three minutes, and immediately sit in a chair. The active part of the test is now completed.
4. At exactly one minute after you complete the test, count your pulse for thirty seconds (see Chapter 3 for pulse-counting instructions) and multiply by 2 to obtain your one-minute pulse recovery score.
5. Determine the rating for your score by consulting the table "Heart Beats per Minute." If you are unable to step for the full three minutes, consider yourself very low in CRE.

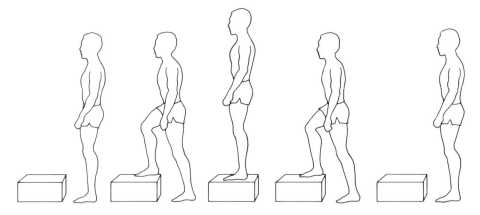

Rating: The scores in the table are for heartbeats per minute, measured 1 minute after completion of the modified step test.

Your score: _____.

Heart Beats per Minute

Age	Very high	High	Moderate	Low	Very low
Female					
10–19	Below 82	82–90	92–96	98–102	Above 102
20–29	Below 82	82–86	88–92	94–98	Above 98
30–39	Below 82	82–88	90–94	96–98	Above 98
40–49	Below 82	82–86	88–96	98–102	Above 102
Over 50	Below 86	86–92	94–98	100–104	Above 104
Male					
10–19	Below 72	72–76	78–82	84–88	Above 88
20–29	Below 72	72–78	80–84	86–92	Above 92
30–39	Below 76	76–80	82–86	88–92	Above 92
40–49	Below 78	78–82	84–88	90–94	Above 94
Over 50	Below 80	80–84	86–90	92–96	Above 96

Assessing your modified step test score: If you are sedentary, your score will probably be around 100 or above, no matter what your age. Conversely, if you're exceptionally fit, your score will be below that of someone your age who is less fit. If your score on the modified step test is well below 100—falling within the very high or high rating—you have high CRE. Chances are you regularly do some activity that enhances CRE. Keep it up. A moderate or low rating indicates there is room for improvement in CRE. If your score falls within the very low rating, then a regular CRE program could make a big difference. Chapter 3 can help you plan a program to increase your CRE, should you so choose. To determine how you're progressing on a CRE program, you may want to use the modified step test on a regular basis. If so, remember to test yourself in the same way and under the same conditions (in the same general health, at the same time of day, at the same interval before or after a meal or vigorous activity, etc.).

PROFILE 1-2

PROFILE 1-3

YOUR FITNESS PROFILE 1-3
Taking the 1.5-Mile Run-Walk Test

Objective: To run, walk, or run-walk a distance of 1.5 miles as quickly as possible. *Warning:* Do not take this test if you are ill or have significant risk factors that predispose you to cornary heart disease (i.e., smoking, obesity, high blood pressure, high blood fats, etc.) without checking with your doctor.

Directions:

1. Locate a running track or other area that provides exact measurements of up to 1.5 miles.
2. Have available a stopwatch or a clock with a clearly visible sweep-second hand.
3. Try to cover the distance at a pace that is best for you. Practice your pacing prior to taking the test to avoid going too fast at the outset and becoming prematurely fatigued. It could be helpful to review the model walk-jog programs in Chapter 7 for suggestions on pacing.
4. Avoid strenuous activity on the day of the test.
5. Avoid heavy eating or smoking for up to 3 hours before taking the test.
6. Avoid taking the test under extreme conditions of heat or cold, particularly if you have not been exercising under those conditions.
7. Warm up before taking the test (see pp. 143–146).
8. Cool down after the test (see pp. 143–146).
9. If possible have someone call out your time at various intervals of the test to determine whether your pace is correct.

Rating: In the table, find your age category and the time (in minutes and seconds) it took you to complete the 1.5-mile course.

Your time: _____.

1.5-Mile Run-Walk Test Ratings

Age	Superior	Excellent	Good	Fair	Poor	Very poor
Female						
13–19	Below 11:50	12:29–11:50	14:30–12:30	16:54–14:31	18:30–16:55	Over 18:31
20–29	Below 12:30	13:30–12:30	15:54–13:31	18:30–15:55	19:00–18:31	Over 19:01
30–39	Below 13:00	14:30–13:00	16:30–14:31	19:00–16:31	19:30–19:01	Over 19:31
40–49	Below 13:45	15:55–13:45	17:30–15:56	19:30–17:31	20:00–19:31	Over 20:01
Over 50	Below 14:30	16:30–14:30	19:00–16:31	20:00–19:01	20:30–20:01	Over 20:31
Male						
13–19	Below 8:37	8:37– 9:40	9:41–10:48	10:49–12:10	12:11–15:30	Over 15:31
20–29	Below 9:45	9:45–10:45	10:46–12:00	12:01–14:00	14:01–16:00	Over 16:01
30–39	Below 10:00	10:00–11:00	11:01–12:30	12:31–14:45	14:44–16:30	Over 16:31
40–49	Below 10:30	10:30–11:30	11:31–13:00	13:01–15:35	15:36–17:30	Over 17:31
Over 50	Below 11:00	11:00–12:30	12:31–14:30	14:31–17:00	17:01–19:00	Over 19:01

YOUR FITNESS PROFILE 1-4
Determining Your Body Build

Objective: To determine your body build by measuring your wrist.

Directions: Measure the circumference of your wrist. One easy way to do this is to wrap a string around your wrist and then measure the length against a ruler.

Body Build Measurements

	Small	*Medium*	*Large*
Female	5.5 inches or less	5.6–6.2 inches	6.3 inches or more
Male	6.7 inches or less	6.8–7.4 inches	7.5 inches or more

Rating: Find your measurement on the table above. Determining your body build will help you use the height-weight chart in Appendix A.

Your measurement: _____.

convenient, so many fitness programs rely instead on skinfold calipers to assess body composition. This device measures the amount of fat lying just beneath the skin, where 50 percent of the body's fat is usually located. Mathematical equations convert the skinfold measurements into an estimate of total body fat.

There are many suggested sites for measuring skinfolds. We have selected a two-site test: for men, thigh and subscapula; for women, triceps and suprailiac. If you wish to use this technique, follow the directions in Profile 1-5 and calculate your body-fat percentage using one of the charts. An interpretation of your results follows.

An easier way to estimate body composition—and it works for both men and women—is the pinch test described by Jean Mayer, an authority on overweight. Locate on your body a fold of skin and subcutaneous fat that may be lifted free—between the thumb and forefinger—from the underlying soft tissue and bone. Some of the body areas that can be used for this test are the back of the upper arm, the side of the lower chest, the back just below the shoulder blade, the back of the calf, and the abdomen. Once you've grasped the fold of skin, do your best to measure it. Mayer explains: "In general, the layer beneath the skin should be between one-fourth and one-half inch; the skinfold is a double thickness and should therefore be one-half to one inch. A fold markedly greater than one inch—for example in the back of the arm—indicates excessive body fatness; one markedly thinner than one-half inch, abnormal thinness."

But the easiest test of all is the mirror test, which can help you estimate body fat. Mayer suggests that you simply look at yourself naked in a mirror. "If you *look* fat, you probably *are* fat," he notes.

Muscular Strength

Your ability to lift a heavy suitcase or bag of groceries gives you a very rough idea of muscular strength. If you experience difficulty removing an ordinary lid from a jar, say, you may lack *minimal* muscular strength. To undertake an assessment of your precise muscular strength could mean comprehensive testing of the body's major muscle groups—a time-consuming process requiring expensive equipment that's not widely available. Such a procedure would be impractical as well as unnecessary for routine self-assessment. Instead, you can settle for a test of grip strength, involving a single muscle group but one that correlates well with tests of general body strength. The most accurate way to test grip strength is by means of a hand dynamometer (see Profile 1-6 and Figure 1-3).

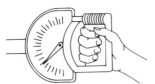

FIGURE 1-3   Hand dynamometer.

Muscular Endurance

Your level of muscular strength is somewhat dependent on your muscular endurance. For example, it takes a certain amount of strength to lift a suitcase, but it takes a certain amount of muscular endurance to hold it off the floor for five minutes. If your muscles usually feel sore a day or two after you go hiking or row a boat, you may be low in muscular endurance. If you tend to talk a lot about your "aching muscles," you may want to focus on improving your muscular endurance.

Sit-ups are commonly used to measure the muscular endurance of the abdominal muscles, and push-ups are used to measure the shoulders, chest, and arms. Following the directions in Profile 1-7, see how many sit-ups you can do in sixty seconds and the number of consecutive push-ups you can complete correctly. Then compare your score with the ratings in the following tables. These ratings are only estimates, but they can be useful in your self-assessment.

Flexibility

Flexibility—how limber you are—encompasses the ability to move a joint through its normal range of motion. To walk up a flight of stairs, for example, you need some flexibility in the hips, knees, and ankles. Flexibility is also related to strength. Muscles contain stretch receptors that help control muscle contractions. When your muscles are too tight, the stretch receptors fire prematurely and cause muscles to be weaker than they normally would be.

Good trunk flexibility may help protect you against low-back pain, which can be related, in part, to tightness of the hamstring muscles (located in the back of the thighs), hips, and lower back. As with muscular strength and endurance, overall flexibility cannot be readily assessed by a single test. One measure of flexibility that can be particularly useful is described in Profile 1-8, which shows you how to evaluate your ability to bend your trunk forward.

ASSESSING YOUR FITNESS

Once you've completed the self-assessment tests, record each score and rating in Profile 1-9 on page 26. This will provide a summary of results, which should help you set some fitness goals for yourself.

SETTING GOALS

With the fitness assessment summary now completed, you may want to set only a general goal—to promote your overall physical fitness by concentrating on the particular components that seem to be most in need of improvement. Or, like many of our students, you may want to cope with a specific health problem or achieve a specific fitness goal.

YOUR FITNESS PROFILE 1-5
Methods for Assessing Body Composition

Using Skinfold Calipers

Objective: To accurately measure the amount of fat located under the skin.

Directions:

1. Have someone trained in the use of skinfold calipers measure you.
2. Take each measurement on the right side of the body.
3. Pinch a fold of skin between the thumb and forefinger. Do not include any muscle tissue in your grasp.
4. Place the contact surfaces of the calipers about ¼ inch below the tips of the pinching fingers.
5. While pinching the skin, permit the contact surfaces to close slowly to ensure that enough pressure is exerted to hold the skinfold.
6. Take readings to the nearest half millimeter.
7. Repeat the measurements until two consecutive measurements match.
8. Skinfold sites for women:
   a. *Suprailiac:* Pinch the skinfold at an angle above the right hip bone.

      Your measurement _____.
   b. *Triceps:* Pinch a vertical skinfold on the back of the arm midway between the shoulder and elbow. Your arm should hang naturally at your side.

      Your measurement _____.

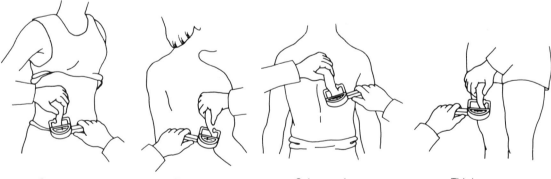

Suprailiac   Triceps   Subscapula   Thigh

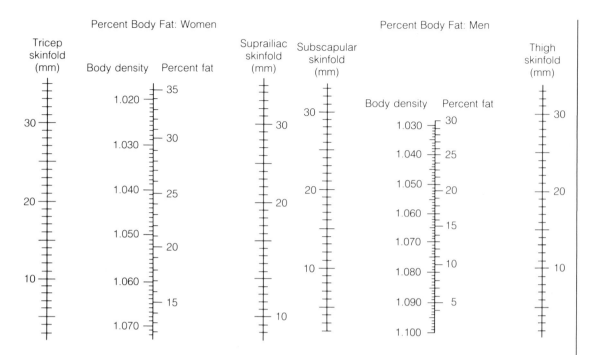

9. Skinfold sites for men:
   a. *Subscapula:* Pinch a diagonal fold just below the lower angle of the right scapula.

   Your measurement _____.
   b. *Thigh:* Pinch a vertical fold midway between the topmost point of the hip bone and the knee cap.

   Your measurement _____.

10. Mark each of your skinfold measurements on the appropriate "percent of body fat" chart. Connect the two marks with a straight line. Read your percent body fat on the middle scale.

Rating: Find your percentage of body fat in the table "Interpreting Body Fat Percentages."

Your percentage: _____.

Interpreting Body Fat Percentages		
	Men (%)	*Women (%)*
Obese	25 and higher	35 and higher
High fat	20–24	30–34
Above average	17–19	25–29
Average	13–16	20–24
Below average	10–12	17–19
Low fat	Below 10	Below 17

(continued)

YOUR FITNESS PROFILE 1-5
Methods for Assessing Body Composition *(continued)*

Body Mass Index

Body mass index (BMI) is a rough measure of body composition. This is a particularly good technique if your only tools for determining body fat are a bathroom scale to measure weight and a tape to measure height. It is a variance of the height-weight table and is based on the concept that a person's weight should be proportional to height. Although this technique has several weaknesses, it is fairly accurate for individuals who do not have an excessive amount of muscle mass.

Objective: To determine proportion of body fat according to individual height. Please note that BMI is not a measure of percent of body fat.

Directions: Using the following chart, place a ruler or other straight edge between the body weight column on the left and the height column on the right and read the BMI from the point where it crosses the center. In the example provided, a 190-pound woman, 65 inches tall (5 foot, 5 inches) would be on the borderline between overweight and obese, with a BMI of 29.5.

Body Mass Index (BMI)

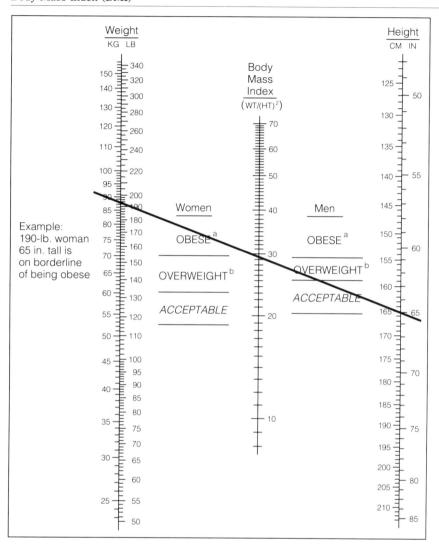

Example:
190-lb. woman
65 in. tall is
on borderline
of being obese

[a] *Obesity:* BMI above 30 kg/m².
[b] *Overweight:* Body mass index (BMI) of 25 to 30 kg/m².
SOURCE: Reprinted with permission from G. A. Bray, 1978, Definitions, measurements and classification of the syndrome of obesity, *International Journal of Obesity* 2:99–112.

Ideal body mass index:

Men should be less than 27.2.
Women should be less than 26.9.

YOUR FITNESS PROFILE 1-6
Taking the Grip-Strength Dynamometer Test

Objective: To assess your grip strength by using a hand dynamometer.

Directions: Hold the dynamometer in one hand (preferably the hand you write with). Squeeze the device as hard as you can; then read your score in pounds (or kilograms) on the dial. Consult the table "Grip Strength" for an interpretation of your grip score. The scores are given in pounds.

Rating: Because there is usually some change in body composition with increased age, scores should be adjusted to reflect an age-related decrease in the ratio of muscle to fat. People over age 50 should, therefore, add about 10 percent to their score.

Your score: _____.

Assessing your grip-strength score: If your score falls within the low or very low rating on the grip test, your overall muscular strength is probably also low or very low. If you choose to improve muscular strength by undertaking a specific exercise program, you are likely to see a dramatic improvement over time in your performance in activities requiring muscular strength. (See Chapter 5 for advice on planning an exercise program in this area.)

Grip Strength (in Pounds)

	Very high	High	Moderate	Low	Very low
Female	Above 89	83–89	56–82	49–55	Below 49
Male	Above 154	136–154	105–135	91–104	Below 91

YOUR FITNESS PROFILE 1-7
Testing Your Muscular Endurance

Objective: To complete as many sit-ups in 60 seconds as possible and to complete as many push-ups or modified push-ups as you possibly can.

Directions:

1. *60-second sit-up* (Note: Don't try this if you have back trouble.): Start with your back flat on the floor and knees bent, feet flat on floor, arms crossed at chest. With feet held down (you'll need someone to assist), perform as many sit-ups as possible in 60 seconds. Touch elbows to your knees or thighs and return to the full starting position each time.

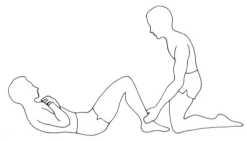

2. *Push-up:* Start in push-up position with arms straight, fingers forward. Lower chest to floor with back straight; then return to starting position. (Note: Many people may have insufficient strength to perform even a single push-up when using the push-up technique described here. The modified push-up allows such people to support themselves with their knees, thus reducing the need for upper-body strength in a test of muscular endurance.)

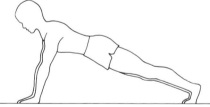

2a. *Modified push-up:* Same as push-up, except that you support yourself with your knees and keep your back straight.

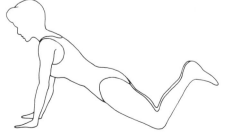

(continued)

YOUR FITNESS PROFILE 1-7
Testing Your Muscular Endurance *(continued)*

Ratings: Your scores are the maximum number of correct sit-ups in 60 seconds and the number of push-ups performed in succession. See the accompanying tables.

Your score for the 60-second sit-up test: _____.

Your score for the push-up or modified push-up test: _____.

Assessing your sit-up test score: This test measures muscular endurance of the abdominal muscles. You can improve a low or very low score by selecting weight training exercises for these muscles.

Assessing your push-up test score: This test evaluates the muscular endurance of your shoulder, arm, and chest muscles. You can improve a low or very low score by weight training exercises for these muscles.

Ratings for 60-Second Sit-up Test

Age	Very high	High	Moderate	Low	Very low
Female					
15–29	Above 43	39–43	33–38	29–32	Below 29
30–39	Above 35	31–35	25–30	21–24	Below 21
40–49	Above 30	26–30	19–25	16–18	Below 16
Over 50	Above 25	21–25	15–20	11–14	Below 11
Male					
15–29	Above 47	43–47	37–42	33–36	Below 33
30–39	Above 39	35–39	29–34	25–28	Below 25
40–49	Above 34	30–34	24–29	20–23	Below 20
Over 50	Above 29	25–29	19–24	15–18	Below 15

Ratings for Push-up and Modified Push-up Tests

Age	Very high	High	Moderate	Low	Very low
Push-up					
15–29	Above 54	45–54	35–44	20–34	Below 20
30–39	Above 44	35–44	25–34	15–24	Below 15
40–49	Above 39	30–39	20–29	12–19	Below 12
Over 50	Above 34	25–34	15–24	8–14	Below 8
Modified push-up					
15–29	Above 48	34–48	17–33	6–16	Below 6
30–39	Above 39	25–39	12–24	4–11	Below 4
40–49	Above 34	20–34	8–19	3–7	Below 3
Over 50	Above 29	15–29	6–14	2–5	Below 2

YOUR FITNESS PROFILE 1-8
Testing Your Trunk Flexibility

Objective: To reach as far forward as possible while sitting with your knees straight.

Directions: Before beginning this test, do some warm-up stretching exercises, such as bending sideways, forward, and backward several times, and rotating your trunk. Warm-ups may not only make it easier to perform the test, they may also help prevent strain or injury. In doing this test and the warm-ups that precede it, make your movements slow and gradual—never fast or jerky. Once warmed up, follow the procedure described below to test your trunk flexibility.

1. Place a box on the floor against a wall.
2. Tape a ruler on the box so that the 4-inch mark is on line with the near edge of the box and the 12-inch mark is farthest from you at the wall end of the box.
3. Sit on the floor with your legs extended so that your heels are about 5 inches apart and your feet are flat against the box.
4. Slowly reach with both hands as far forward as possible. Touch your fingertips to the yardstick and hold this position for about three seconds. Check the yardstick and note the distance you have reached.
5. Try this three times. (Do not attempt to add length by jerking forward.) Your flexibility score is the best of three trials.

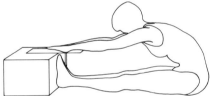

Rating: The scores in the "Trunk Flexibility" table are for the number of inches you reached.

Your score: _____.

Trunk Flexibility (in Inches)

	Very high	*High*	*Moderate*	*Low*	*Very low*
Female	Above 12	10–11	6–9	2–5	Below 2
Male	Above 11	8–10	3–7	1–2	Below 1

Assessing Your Trunk Flexibility Test Score: Although this test is a fair estimate of general flexibility for most people, it does not allow for differences in arm and leg length. Individuals with poor trunk flexibility could attain a good score on the test if they have long arms and short legs. Likewise individuals with short arms and long legs would attain poor scores. Women tend to be more flexible than men, as reflected in the scores listed. If your score on the trunk flexibility test falls within the low or very low rating and you cannot attribute this to short arms or long legs, then you may want to regularly do some of the various hamstring-stretching exercises suggested in the stretching model program in Chapter 7.

YOUR FITNESS PROFILE 1-9
A Summary of Your Fitness

Objective: To summarize the results of the physical fitness self-assessment tests in this chapter.

Directions: After completing Profiles 1-1, 1-2, 1-3, 1-5, 1-6, 1-7, and 1-8, fill in this worksheet to get a rough estimate of how you rate in each of the five components of physical fitness. The comments column provides space for noting any areas that need improvement.

Components of Physical Fitness

Activity index: _____ Estimated level of activity: _____

Components and tests	Results	Rating	Comments
Cardiorespiratory endurance			
Modified step test	_____	_____	_____
1.5-mile run-walk	_____	_____	_____
Body composition Percentage body fat	_____	_____	_____
Pinch test (p. 16)	_____	N/A	_____
Mirror test (p. 16)	_____	N/A	_____
BMI	_____	_____	_____
Muscular strength Grip strength	_____	_____	_____
Muscular endurance 60-second sit-up	_____	_____	_____
Push-up	_____	_____	_____
Modified push-up	_____	_____	_____
Flexibility Trunk flexibility	_____	_____	_____

For the sake of your health you may find you need to improve the way your heart and lungs function. Perhaps you decide it's time to lose weight and tone up some muscles to enhance your appearance. Or you may believe it prudent to keep limber to protect yourself from disabling stiffness in your later years. These goals, of course, are all keyed to specific components of physical fitness. To fortify heart and lungs, you work on cardiorespiratory endurance (CRE). To slim down and firm up, you concentrate on body composition. To be limber, you work on flexibility.

What if you want to get in shape for tennis, increase your stamina, or improve your posture? The appropriate exercise regimen to achieve such goals may not be as clearly keyed to a single component: It may require a combination of more than one component. For example, getting in shape for tennis calls for developing CRE, increasing the strength and muscular endurance of your arms and legs, and improving flexibility.

No matter which approaches to fitness you favor, you may find it helpful to look over Table 1-2. It lists the twenty-seven goals that we have encountered most often together with the fitness components most likely to be strengthened by a program designed to meet each of the goals.

Many common fitness goals, as Table 1-2 indicates, depend for their realization on simultaneously upgrading more than one fitness component. But even if you choose to work on just a single component, such a program would still be likely to improve other components as well. For instance, jogging undertaken primarily to improve your cardiorespiratory condition will probably also improve your body composition and have some effect on the muscular endurance of your legs.

Cardiorespiratory endurance ratings, body fat percentages, and grip test scores tend to be abstract and impersonal concepts. Few of our students initially used terms such as increased CRE or improved body composition to describe their goals. What many hoped for from a fitness regimen was "freedom from backaches," "more stamina," "better muscle tone," and the like. Such goals are readily translatable into fitness components. For example, as noted earlier, an increase in muscular strength and flexibility—especially in the muscles and joints of the lower trunk—could help reduce susceptibility to low-back pain.

Once you have completed the fitness assessment summary, reviewed Table 1-2 for ideas about goals you might like to achieve, and noted which components are most involved in achieving those goals, then you will have a better sense of the specific training program you may want to pursue. Refer to the contents page for the chapters most relevant to your goals.

Improvement in physical fitness may not be the only achievement of those who set fitness goals for themselves. Those who have shared with us their own current fitness programs mentioned intangible by-products of various forms of exercise. Eighteen-year-old Lynne, for example, believes a program of regular jogging has given her "a sense of peace and calm as well as a feeling of personal accomplishment."

Running every day, according to Ted, a 30-year-old clinical psychologist, "is guaranteed to relax me and clear my mind of any disturbing thoughts. It is almost a form of psychotherapy." Kirstan, age 21, says that by pushing herself beyond what she thought she could endure, her exercise program has given her "a whole new image" of herself.

TABLE 1-2   Specific Fitness Goals and Components Involved in Their Achievement

Goals	CRE	Body composition	Muscular strength	Muscular endurance	Flexibility
Recuperate from surgery	✔		✔	✔	✔
Prevent, eliminate, or reduce low-back pain; recover from an orthopedic problem	✔	✔	✔	✔	✔
Make pregnancy and childbirth easier	✔	✔	✔	✔	✔
Eliminate or reduce breathlessness brought on by climbing stairs, etc.	✔	✔		✔	
Increase stamina in such activities as jogging, swimming, dancing, bicycling, long walks	✔	✔		✔	
Increase resistance to muscle fatigue	✔		✔	✔	
Increase muscular effectiveness for daily tasks, sports activities			✔	✔	✔
Become more muscular; firm up muscle tone		✔	✔	✔	
Reduce risk of circulatory and respiratory system disorders	✔	✔			
Lower high blood pressure	✔	✔			
Help to improve control of diabetes	✔	✔			
Lower cholesterol and/or triglyceride levels	✔	✔			
Increase high-density lipoprotein cholesterol	✔	✔			
Reduce discomfort from arthritis		✔			✔
Prevent, eliminate, or reduce muscle and/or joint injury			✔		✔
Decrease muscle soreness due to physical activity				✔	✔
Have more energy at the end of a day's activities	✔			✔	
Improve posture				✔	✔
Reduce menstrual discomfort			✔		✔
Prevent heart attack at an early age	✔	✔			
Lower the resting heart rate	✔				
Reduce asthmatic discomfort during exercise	✔				
Increase range of movement and become more limber					✔
Reduce discomfort from tension					✔
Improve fit of clothes		✔			
Lose or gain weight		✔			
Look trimmer by reducing the girth of waist, hips, thighs, arms		✔			

We have received hundreds of testimonials noting that since undertaking a regular fitness regimen, people sleep better, eat more sensibly, work harder. Many say they have greater enthusiasm, feel better about themselves, and are less jittery or irritable; quite a few say their sex life has improved. These positive side effects of improved physical fitness are difficult to explain, and they are harder to predict than improvement in the measurable components. Although no one can guarantee that becoming physically fit by following an exercise program will enhance the quality of life, many of our students thought it did.

What physical fitness training can do is make some distinct, measurable improvements in one or more of the five components. These in turn can help you achieve some of the fitness goals you have set for yourself. Success can't be guaranteed, and it certainly isn't easy to achieve in any case. But for many people, physical fitness is definitely worth a try. And trying for it can even be fun.

2

Physical Fitness Training Principles

After you've read this chapter, you will be able to:

Explain how progressive overload can result in training effects.

Identify how the specificity of an activity can achieve particular fitness goals.

Define *intensity of exercise, duration of exercise,* and *frequency of exercise.*

Apply exercise intensity, duration, and frequency to provide progressive overload.

The human body has an extraordinary ability to respond to the physical demands placed on it if sound training principles are used and the level of demands is escalated slowly. In a graduated program, the muscles involved progressively increase in strength and endurance with each small increment of activity. As the individual muscle fibers increase in size, the muscles gain in strength. This process, known as *hypertrophy,* occurs slowly as the demands on muscles gradually increase. Abrupt increases in activity levels, however, could cause tendon and muscle injuries.

PROGRESSIVE OVERLOAD

If you have never lifted anything heavier than a 10-pound bag of groceries, you may not find it so easy to pick up one end of a sofa, let alone carry it up two flights of stairs. But professional movers would probably not find it difficult. Undoubtedly, they have become quite accustomed to carrying heavy furniture. The weight would be less of a strain for them because they lift heavy loads daily.

When you make demands such as this on your body, its first response is to mobilize its resources to accomplish the greater work load. The muscles involved will strain somewhat to accomplish the task; heart rate, breathing, and blood flow to those muscles will all increase sharply. But with repetition of the activity over a period of time, the body becomes adapted to the increased work load. The heart, lungs, and muscles function more efficiently, accomplishing the same work with less exertion.

This kind of experience—adaptation of the body to new demands—results from *progressive overload,* the first of two fundamental principles of sound fitness training. (We discuss the second, *specificity,* below.) Progressive overload can be achieved by increasing one or more of three factors: intensity, duration, and frequency. To lift heavier packages in a stockroom job means that the *intensity* of the activity has increased. If you also put in overtime, you increase the *duration.* And working six days a week instead of five increases the *frequency.* As your body adapts

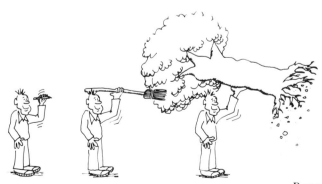

Progressive overload.

to the new demands, you acquire a new level of competence and comfort. Last week's exertion becomes today's comfortable work load. Of course, if you reduce your level of activity, the opposite occurs: Your body adjusts to a lower level of competency and strength, and yesterday's acceptable work load becomes next week's overload.

If you ever had an arm or a leg in a cast or were confined to bed after surgery, you no doubt recall how your body adapted to the lack of movement. The size and strength of the affected muscles atrophied, and there was a general decline in strength, endurance, and flexibility. As you recovered, you probably applied progressive overload even if you didn't have professional guidance for your rehabilitation. When the cast was removed or when strict bed rest was no longer necessary, you most likely arranged your day so that you would avoid any excessive effort. Perhaps you limited your stair climbing to once a day, took a nap after lunch, and went to bed early in the evening. When you returned to your regular routine, it was probably only part time at first. Gradually you extended the range of your activities until eventually you were able to resume everything you had formerly been able to do.

Your recovery was geared to a slow but steady restoration of impaired muscular strength, endurance, and flexibility. By progressively demanding more and more from your body, you made use of your body's normal ability to adapt in time to new demands. Sound physical fitness programs, like therapeutic programs, are based on the body's self-protective capacity for adaptation. If you start with a work load at, or only slightly above, your ordinary level of fitness and then very slowly and steadily increase the work load, you will make slow but steady improvement in your fitness level.

The positive adaptations your body makes to new and increasingly rigorous demands are known as *training effects*. For example, the training effects of a program for cardiorespiratory endurance (CRE) would include reduced heart rate while at rest and during activity and also breathing more comfortably during activity. The training effects of a program to improve body composition would include an increase in the size and weight of skeletal muscles and a decrease in body fat. In short, training effects are the benefits you get from a regular exercise program, practiced in accordance with the training principle of progressive overload.

When overloading becomes excessive, however, there may be unpleasant and even painful reactions. Starting out at too demanding a level of activity or going too soon to the next level usually results in aches, pains, and discouragement.

If you experience symptoms such as the following, the cause is probably excessive overload:

- Rapid heart rate—at the level experienced during the activity—persisting five to ten minutes after the activity has stopped
- Fatigue continuing twenty-four hours after the activity has stopped
- Muscle soreness (charley horse or feeling muscle-bound)

If you gradually increase the demands you make on yourself when you begin a fitness program, you can avoid problems such as these. A little overload goes a long way. The watchword should be, "Train, don't strain." Start with a slight overload and increase it steadily to get your training effects with little or no discomfort.

SPECIFICITY

Hand in hand with progressive overload goes *specificity,* the second fundamental principle of sound fitness training. Your fitness program must be specifically designed to meet your goals. You need quite different programs to get in shape for varsity basketball than you do for weekend tennis doubles, neither of which requires total fitness. Exercises to develop arm strength aren't the same as those used for rehabilitation after a heart attack. The principle of specificity is that only those body systems that are stressed by an exercise program will achieve the beneficial effects of fitness training.

Sometimes, of course, an exercise program may be inappropriate for a particular goal. Take, for example, Frank. "Throughout most of my life, I've been rather heavy around the middle." Frank described himself as 5 feet 8 inches, with a 40-inch waist when he first turned to exercise. At a friend's suggestion, Frank did "lots of sit-ups—morning, noon, and night" for three months. Even though he was doing hundreds a day, his waist size didn't change, and he finally gave up. However, a month or so later, he "read that aerobic activities like running or cycling are supposed to be excellent for weight loss. I took up cycling, riding an hour a day, five days a week, and attempted to control my eating. After a few months I had to add some new notches to my belt—down to a 38." A year later, he reported, he had a 34-inch waist.

For every fitness goal, there is a variety of appropriate activities to choose from. Your choice should take into consideration such factors as how an activity is paced, the level of skill and fitness prerequisite required, intensity, duration, and frequency. Other aspects to consider—the degree of sociality involved in an activity, its convenience, its cost, your current level of health, your age, and your interests—are covered in Chapter 13.

Some individuals prefer to alternate two or more activities to improve a single component of fitness. Caryn, for example, works hard to improve her CRE by jogging, swimming, and skipping rope. She feels that this approach reduces overuse injuries and keeps her from becoming bored. This method of choosing more than one activity is called *cross training*.

Cross training is epitomized by athletes who train for and compete in the triathlon, a single event consisting of swimming, bicycling, and running, each for a long distance.

How an Activity Is Paced

Pace can be an important consideration. If it is up to you to set the pace, there may be no problem: You can go at the rate necessary to maintain your heart rate within your exercise benefit zone (see discussion beginning on page 52). But if others are involved, your benefit from an activity can be affected. You will need to consider, say, other participants' skill levels, the demands of an activity leader, or the need to keep up with other participants.

Level of Skill and Fitness Prerequisite

If your activity index is low, or if you performed poorly in one or two of the self-assessment tests in Chapter 1, you should choose activities that are self-paced and appropriate for your particular level of fitness. Some activities require such complex skills or such a high level of fitness that they may not be practical for anyone beginning a fitness program. Be sure to choose activities that you can perform with enough skill to achieve the goals you have set for yourself. You do not need to have athletic skills, for example, to improve your cardiorespiratory endurance with a jogging program. But to improve CRE by playing tennis, you need enough skill to sustain a rally long enough to achieve and maintain an elevated heart rate.

DESIGNING AN EXERCISE PROGRAM

Below are some general guidelines to help you decide on a suitable exercise program. Detailed information about various exercise programs and activities is found in Chapter 7 and Appendix B. Whatever your fitness goals and whatever your choice of exercise, the cornerstones of your program will be progressive overload and specificity.

By making use of the information in Chapter 7 and Appendix B to help you select an activity to achieve a particular goal, you are applying the principle of specificity. You may find yourself juggling variables and weighing personal priorities as you consider all the criteria before you make your choice. For example, you may end up selecting an activity not so much because it's interesting and enjoyable but because it's convenient. Fortunately, no selection need be permanent. You can always change activities to meet changing needs and interests. (And that is a good reason to avoid making too great a financial commitment at the beginning of a fitness program.)

Once you have decided on an appropriate exercise program, you should begin to apply the principle of progressive overload. Ask yourself three questions: How hard should I exercise? How long should I keep at it in each session? How often should I do it? In other words, you need to attain training effects by adjusting the type, intensity, duration, and frequency of your exercise sessions.

How Hard?

The *intensity* at which you start a specific program depends on how fit you are. But no matter what your current level of fitness, improvement will come only as your body adapts to the increased demands you place on it. Suppose you swim one lap of a 25-yard pool in one minute but you need to rest for two minutes before you can swim another lap. That effort would represent your beginning level of intensity. Then suppose your program calls for swimming every other day. After a few weeks, you will find you can swim the first lap faster and begin the second lap after a shorter rest period. What has happened is that you have increased your intensity (faster lap time and shorter rest period) as your body responds to the new demands placed on it.

Similarly, if you are a jogger beginning an exercise program to improve CRE, you could increase intensity by quickening your pace or by running uphill. If you are riding a stationary bicycle to improve body composition, you can intensify your effort by increasing the resistance against which you pedal or by pedaling faster. If you are a weight trainer working for muscular strength and endurance, you can put more weight on the bar or increase the number of repetitions. If you are doing calisthenics to increase flexibility, you could raise the intensity by stretching farther.

In establishing your beginning level of intensity, always remember it is best to be conservative. You should not feel that you are working hard when you exercise. Be patient; you can increase your work load gradually as your body becomes conditioned. During CRE activity, your heart rate serves as your guide to how fast you should increase your work load. During muscular strength and muscular endurance training, it will be the amount of resistance or the number of repetitions you can manage. In flexibility workouts, the extent of your stretch will be the criterion.

How Long?

The *duration* of your exercise session will depend in part on its intensity. In general, the duration of the activity should be between twenty and sixty minutes. The less demanding the activity, the longer the session can be. If you jog, you could run for a longer time by slowing your pace or you could run for a shorter time at a faster pace. In weight training, if you increase the load, you will probably have to reduce the number of repetitions until you adapt to the greater weight.

But when you have limited time for exercise it can be useful to increase the intensity to make the most of the time available. A good tennis player, for example, will get more training effects from forty-five minutes of vigorous singles with an equally skilled opponent than from two hours of doubles against less skilled competitors.

Because intensity and duration are so closely related, you will often have to adjust one to the other. For example, high-intensity activity will usually be limited in duration because fatigue sets in more quickly. If you want to work at high intensity, you can compensate for this to some extent by using a method of training called *interval training*. It involves alternating brief rest periods with bouts of exercise. A jogger might alternate one minute of walking with two minutes of jogging. A rope skipper might break a session with a one-minute rest period every two minutes or with two-minute intervals of reduced intensity—stretching exercises, say, or calisthenics. A swimmer might take a rest from the crawl by doing the sidestroke for a lap or two. To increase training effects with interval training, you can shorten the resting period or step up the intensity.

How Often?

The *frequency* of your workouts depends on such factors as how much time you have available, your goals, and the time span in which you hope to achieve them. You should try to train three to five days per week. Remember that physical fitness is only temporary. You may begin to lose some training effects as soon as two or three days after a workout. Obviously, then, weekend exercise is not enough. Daily workouts may be somewhat more beneficial than a session every other day, but for a general fitness program, an every-other-day schedule seems to offer the best return for the time invested. If weight loss is a goal, you will probably need five or more exercise periods a week to use up the calories your program calls for. Whatever your fitness goals, however, once you have achieved your desired fitness level, you can probably maintain it with fewer exercise periods a week.

Table 2-1 illustrates how the training principles of specificity and progressive overload can be used to increase fitness levels for each of the five components.

TABLE 2-1   Applying Training Principles to Fitness Components

To benefit one or more of the five components of physical fitness, an activity must take into account the two fundamental training principles. To illustrate specificity, a sample of appropriate activities for each component is listed below. To define progressive overload, the requirements of intensity, duration, and frequency are given for each of the components. Note that for muscular endurance two approaches are offered: calisthenics and weight training; intensity and duration differ for the two.

Fitness components	Examples of specificity	Progressive overload		
		Intensity	Duration	Frequency
Cardiorespiratory endurance (see Chapter 3)	Bicycling, jogging, rope skipping, swimming, walking	Increase pace as heart rate permits; maintain heart rate in EBZ (see p. 53)	Gradually prolong exercise time; 20 minutes is minimum for training effects	At least every other day
Body composition (see Chapter 4)	Bicycling, jogging, swimming, walking	Increase pace as heart rate permits	Gradually prolong exercise time; 30 minutes is minimum for training effects	At least every other day; aim for 5 days a week if goal is to reduce body fat and/or weight
Muscular strength (see Chapter 5)	Weight training	Use barbells to perform 6 repetitions; at 10 repetitions, increase weight	Increase by repeating each set of 6–10 repetitions	At least every other day
Muscular endurance (see Chapter 5)	Calisthenics	Increase difficulty of exercises	Increase by repeating each set of repetitions	At least every other day
	Weight training	Use barbells to perform 15–25 repetitions; at 25 repetitions, increase weight	Increase by repeating each set of 15–25 repetitions	At least every other day
Flexibility (see Chapter 5)	Calisthenics, modern dance, yoga	Use moderate force to stretch joints	Gradually prolong stretching time for each exercise from 10 up to 60 seconds	At least every other day

HOW TO GET STARTED

If your current level of activity is low, you should start out very slowly. Begin at a starting level of one of the model programs (see Chapter 7). Don't step up the pace until you find that your muscles have adjusted to the new demands placed on them, and even then progress should be slow. You may decide to begin with a model walking or jogging program. After several weeks or more on the model program, you may wish to switch to one of the activities described in Appendix B. Or you may want to experiment with a mix of several different activities once you have moved beyond the initial stage of conditioning.

No matter which activity you select, it should always be preceded and followed by warm-up and cool-down routines (see stretching model program in Chapter 7). Plan to give at least ten minutes to warming up, including stretching, before you begin a workout. And cool down or recover by tapering off your exercise for at least five minutes after the workout.

No matter how pressed you are for time, don't skip the warm-up period. It serves several important functions. It can prevent or reduce muscle and joint injuries and soreness. If you are working on improving CRE, a warm-up period can prepare your cardiorespiratory system gradually for the high level of stress that exercise may place on it. And it can help you get psychologically ready for your exercise session.

Stretching—which should be a slow, easy, gradual process—can be particularly useful as a prelude to such activities as walking and jogging, which require the constant repetition of a limited range of motion of the hamstring, calf, and low-back muscles. Unless stretched, these muscles may tighten and thus cause a variety of discomforts and problems that could put a temporary—or even permanent—end to exercise.

The cool-down period, as the term implies, is a time of reduced activity at the end of a workout. If you have been running, for example, you would reduce the intensity of your activity by slowing to a walk for the last quarter-mile or so. During the cool-down period, your body returns to normal, with heart rate, breathing, and circulation all restored to near pre-exercise levels. With a cool-down period you are less likely to suffer nausea or lightheadedness, which can sometimes occur after strenuous

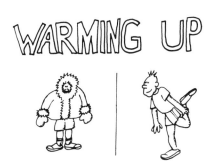

INCORRECT   CORRECT

Warm-up and cool-down routines are vital to a sound exercise program.

exercise. Some people like to repeat the stretching exercises once over lightly as part of the cool-down, and they should now seem much easier and more relaxing than before the workout. Stretching out again at the end of the workout is a good way to prevent muscle tightness and cramping.

In Chapters 7 and 13, we offer suggestions about how best to launch an exercise program. We also suggest various strategies to help you keep going should some of your enthusiasm for exercise begin to fade.

Overenthusiasm can also be a problem. Crash exercising is something like crash dieting: In an excess of zeal or despair—or perhaps some of each—people set impossible goals and go overboard in an effort to achieve them. Instant fitness cannot be achieved, and in the aftermath, people often become so discouraged they lapse into a condition even worse than the one they were in before the crash program. But if you set realistic goals, select activities that can help you achieve them, and work gradually and steadily, you are likely to succeed.

3

Cardiorespiratory Endurance

After you've read this chapter, you will be able to:

Differentiate between aerobic and anaerobic activities.

Identify the cardiorespiratory training effects of aerobic activities.

Determine your exercise benefit zone (EBZ) to guide the intensity of your own cardiorespiratory endurance exercise program.

Accurately take your pulse to measure heart rate.

Determine your optimal exercise duration and frequency to achieve cardiorespiratory fitness goals.

Recognize the relationship of calories used per week during aerobic exercise to various levels of cardiorespiratory endurance (CRE).

Identify how various training programs are used to develop CRE.

Recognize the risk factors of coronary heart disease (CHD).

Identify the role of aerobic exercise in heart health.

Almost anywhere nowadays you're likely to see people running—in track shorts or sweat suits, alone or in pairs or in packs, on roads or sidewalks or cinderpaths. Some smile, some chat with each other, and some grimly chug ahead. They come in all ages and sizes. Among our students, runners, joggers, and walkers outnumber those who exercise by bicycling, rope skipping, and swimming. All these activities are effective ways to achieve cardiorespiratory endurance (CRE).

For some people, exercise is more than just a routine. Norman wrote, "I have almost reached the point where I psychologically need the daily run." One 30-year-old woman reported that her ballet classes "relieve all tensions of the day." Wendy said, "I started by walking to campus and back. . . . Then I became addicted. . . . Even in six inches of snow and thirty below."

Such zeal is, of course, not universal; but deep enjoyment is widespread. Julie, for example, reported that her aerobic dancing class "is the best part of my day." Stan wrote that running provided "a refreshing oasis in a superficial, flashy, image-seeking society."

Some runners take another path. They measure out their miles with little or no enjoyment, running only because they think they should. Seventy-year-old Helen found it "a terrible bore." Nevertheless, she expects to "keep running for another ten years," because otherwise she fears she would "melt away in a chair." Similarly, Juan wrote, "I force myself to keep going year after year. . . . I jog at 6 A.M., before I am awake enough to realize how much I hate it."

Love it, like it, or loathe it, these people spend hour after hour exercising out of a deep conviction that it will benefit them. Many said that they began exercising to overcome their lack of stamina. Most reported that they achieved good results. They claim that their energy levels have increased, they are sleeping better, feel more relaxed, suffer fewer headaches, have less insomnia, and get fewer colds than they did before they started exercising. They smoke less, drink less, and control their weight more easily. Although it is difficult to prove that exercise caused all the good results, many of the reported benefits of regular training are consistent with increased CRE.

In Chapter 1 we defined CRE as the ability to perform moderately strenuous activity over an extended period of time—to swim continuously for twenty minutes, say, or to walk two miles in a half hour. The terms CRE and aerobic fitness can be used interchangeably. Running a mile depends primarily on aerobic fitness—the ability of the cardiorespiratory system to deliver the regular, steady supply of oxygen required by the heart and other muscles.

An *aerobic* activity is any sustained, moderately strenuous effort carried on at an intensity level just high enough to let the heart and lungs keep pace with the increased need for oxygen required by the working muscles.

Sudden rigorous activity, such as sprinting—for a bus or a touchdown—is usually *anaerobic*.

High-intensity exercise uses fast-twitch muscle fibers, which are stronger and faster than slow-twitch muscle fibers used during aerobic activities. Fast-twitch fibers do not use as much oxygen as slow-twitch fibers and rely on the rapid breakdown of carbohydrates for fuel. Carbohydrates are important fuels for high-intensity exercise because they provide energy to the muscles much more rapidly than fats or proteins.

During intense exercise, carbohydrates are used rapidly and a substance called lactic acid is produced at a rapid rate. Lactic acid is believed to be involved in fatigue and, until recently, was believed to be a waste product. Many recent studies have shown that it is an important fuel at rest and during exercise used by most tissues in the body, particularly by the heart, liver, and kidneys. During heavy exercise, lactic acid accumulates in the blood because the rate at which it is produced exceeds the rate the tissues can use it as a fuel.

Training increases your ability to use lactic acid as a fuel. The way this occurs is complex but elegant. Glycogen, the principal carbohydrate used by muscle during exercise, is the critical fuel for exercise, but the body's supply is limited. Training prevents lactic acid buildup by providing the muscles with an increased capacity to use lactic acid as a fuel and prevents glycogen depletion by allowing the muscles to use more fats.

A 100-yard dash is almost purely anaerobic. A marathon is almost entirely aerobic. Most exercise, however, combines aerobic activity with anaerobic spurts. A mile run, for example, is mainly aerobic. But in the home stretch, the miler calls upon fast-twitch muscles to sprint faster, take the lead, and fend off challengers. The well-trained miler must have a high-capacity cardiorespiratory system and a metabolic system capable of using lactic acid as a fuel (see box on pp. 42–43). High-intensity anaerobic activity, such as sprinting, can be tolerated for only short periods of time.

If your anaerobic reserves come into play at a relatively low level of activity and you become fatigued and exhausted easily, you probably have low CRE and low aerobic capacity. If your CRE is sufficient to sustain a high level of activity, then you probably have high aerobic capacity as well as high CRE. *Aerobic capacity* is the maximum amount of oxygen your cardiorespiratory system can deliver to the muscles during the most strenuous activity you can do.

You can increase your aerobic capacity by undertaking a regular CRE training program. How much you can improve depends on factors such as your age, initial level of fitness, and the intensity, duration, and frequency of the training program you select. (To benefit CRE, an exercise must involve the body's largest muscle groups—the legs, including thighs, and the back.) For competitive athletes, there seems to be an inherent limit in aerobic capacity that they encounter within two years after beginning CRE training.* (Reaching a plateau on various occasions during training is also common and should not be confused with reaching a built-in limit.)

---

*Despite this limit, athletes can continue to improve their performance in long-distance events. They can often better their previous records by performing for longer periods of time at a greater percentage of their aerobic capacity. For example, long-distance runners who have reached their inherent limit and therefore cannot expect any further increase in aerobic capacity may still become capable of improving their time in running a race. Further CRE training may enable them to maintain a pace in running a marathon, for example, at a higher percentage of aerobic capacity for a longer period during the race. Indeed, some champion-class marathoners can run at more than 80 percent of their aerobic capacity for a full twenty-six miles—a feat that results in improved competitive time.

OXYGEN AND ENERGY PRODUCTION

We often take our breathing, heart beat, urine formation, and other life-sustaining functions for granted. Yet these vital processes require energy even when a person is at rest or asleep. The body forms and stores energy by means of complicated metabolic reactions requiring the breakdown of carbohydrates, fats, and proteins. These reactions require oxygen. While fuels are stored in the body, oxygen must be continuously obtained from the environment and delivered to the tissues.

When you inhale, oxygen enters your lungs, passes through the thin membranes that line the tiny air sacs of the lungs, and enters the bloodstream. There it combines with hemoglobin in the red blood cells and is carried through the bloodstream to all the cells of the body. When the oxygen in the cells has been consumed, carbon dioxide is picked up by the blood and delivered to the lungs and the kidneys for elimination from the body. With every exhaled breath, we return carbon dioxide and water to the air—along with any unused oxygen. It is therefore possible that cardiorespiratory endurance can be adversely affected by a lower concentration of oxygen in the inhaled air (as at high altitudes), by certain lung diseases that interfere with the transport of oxygen into the bloodstream, or by anemia (a decrease in the number of red blood cells).

Getting oxygen from the air into the bloodstream is the function of the entire respiratory system from the nose to the tiny air sacs of the lungs. Distribution of the oxygen to the cells of the body is the job of the cardiovascular system—the heart and the blood vessels. The heart is composed almost entirely of specialized muscle fibers. It contracts more or less rhythmically and steadily about 90,000 times each day. Each time the heart muscle contracts, blood is pumped out of the chambers of the heart into the arteries. During relaxation (between beats) oxygen-poor blood enters the right side of the heart from the veins of the body. From there it is pumped into the lungs to receive oxygen from the inhaled air. This blood, now rich in oxygen, returns to the left side of the heart, from which it is pumped into the arteries for delivery to all of the body's organs and tissues.

Just how much oxygen you need is directly related to your current level of activity. When you are resting or sleeping, your activity level is minimal. Because less energy is required, less oxygen is consumed. Your breathing rate is slow and shallow and, therefore, less air is inhaled. Your heart pumps more slowly, and oxygenated blood is circulated through your system at a slower rate. During exercise, your oxygen consumption goes up because functions requiring oxygen increase. The ultimate exercise intensity you can reach is determined by the amount of oxygen you can consume and your ability to manage metabolic acids.

During recovery from exercise, oxygen consumption continues to be elevated above normal resting values. In the past this excess post-exercise oxygen consumption was thought to be due to the accumulation of lactic acid that occurred because not enough oxygen was available to the body during exercise. The excess post-exercise oxygen consumption was called *oxygen debt*. The real cause of increased post-exercise oxygen consumption is not due to repaying a debt caused by insufficient oxygen delivery

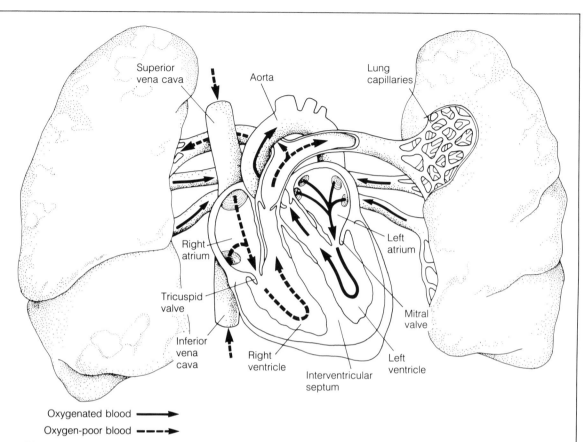

The cardiorespiratory system. Oxygen-poor blood enters the right side of the heart through two large veins. It goes through the two chambers and is pumped into the lungs, where capillaries absorb oxygen from inhaled air. The now oxygen-rich blood flows into the left side of the heart, where it is pumped into the arteries that return it to the rest of the body.

during exercise, but is due to the disturbance of the body's delicate metabolic balance. Exercise causes a rise in metabolic rate, tissue temperature, and hormone secretions and disturbs delicate cellular membranes. All of these factors cause oxygen consumption to increase after exercise. What about lactic acid, the so-called culprit in this process? It is used as a fuel during recovery, in much the same way that blood sugar and fats are used. To lessen the sensation of fatigue caused by metabolic acids, increase your ability to use them during exercise through training.

CARDIORESPIRATORY TRAINING EFFECTS

Marta was anxious to take a college backpacking course and began a walking/jogging program to help her keep up with her fellow students. At first, walking a mile exhausted her. After several weeks she was able to alternate her walking with intervals of slow jogging. Soon she was doing more jogging, with intervals of walking. After two months, she could jog two miles with only brief walking intervals. Then she stalled. Weeks went by without any improvement. She wondered whether she would ever be able to jog the entire two-mile distance without having to walk at all. Finally it happened, during her fifth month on the program. "We were jogging on a nearby quarter-mile track, talking as usual," she reported, "when I suddenly realized that we were finishing the sixth lap and I hadn't walked yet." She wasn't panting and her heart wasn't pounding.

Marta's cardiorespiratory endurance had improved enough to increase her aerobic capacity significantly. The change had come from improvements in many elements of her cardiorespiratory system. The heart of the matter, of course, is the heart itself, the body's pump. The adult heart contracts from 50 to 100 times a minute with an average of 70 contractions per minute, depending on factors such as sex (6 to 8 beats higher in women) and occupation. The number of systoles (heart contractions) per minute is defined as the *heart rate.* The amount of blood pumped out of the heart by each systole is called the *stroke volume,* which varies in normal adults from 70 to 100 milliliters at rest. The stroke volume is usually larger in a slower beating heart, because a slow heart rate allows more time between beats (the diastolic time interval) for the heart to fill with blood. *Cardiac output* is the total amount of blood the heart pumps in one minute. It is computed by multiplying stroke volume by heart rate. At rest, the heart pumps about five liters of blood per minute.

There was no documentation of Marta's marked improvement in physical fitness. Her heart rate had not been checked, and her stroke volume and cardiac output had not been estimated at the beginning of her training program and again when she had achieved her two-mile running goal. Nor had she been weighed and measured and some of her blood chemistries studied. The improvement was real, nevertheless, and reflects specific training effects—positive adaptations of her body to progressively increasing demands. These included an increase in the size and strength of the heart muscle, a reduction in heart rate both at rest and during activity, an increase in stroke volume and cardiac output, and a reduction in the time it takes for the heart to return to resting levels after exercise.

At one time there was concern about "athlete's heart," an enlarged heart shadow found on chest X rays of some athletes. It was thought that a heart of greater than normal size and volume was synonymous with a heart enlarged by disease; therefore many athletes with such X rays were told to curtail their activities. It is now understood that athlete's heart is due to the increased size of the ventricular chamber as well as increased development of the heart muscle.* And muscular development is

---

* An enlarged heart shadow on chest X rays can take several shapes, only one of which represents the so-called athlete's heart. When doubt exists about whether an enlarged heart shadow warrants further exami-

a beneficial training effect of a CRE program, resulting in a strengthened heart with a slow beat.

CRE training results in an increase in the body's blood volume (the total amount of blood) and in plasma volume (plasma is the fluid in which blood cells are carried). The larger total blood volume reflects a small increase in the number of red cells, which results in an improved oxygen-carrying capacity. The increase in blood plasma improves your ability to regulate body temperature and makes the blood less thick, enabling it to flow more easily and rapidly through the circulatory system.

We know that the capability of the circulatory system to deliver oxygen is also influenced by the health of the arteries. The health of the coronary arteries, those that feed the heart, is particularly critical. Coronary heart disease (CHD) and its relationship to heart attacks is the greatest single cause of death in the United States.

The sudden deaths caused by heart attacks are not really so sudden, but rather are usually the end result of a process that began early in life. With age, the flexible walls of the coronary arteries gradually become clogged with fatty substances that cause them to harden and narrow, thereby reducing the blood flow and oxygen supply to the heart. This narrowing process is called atherosclerosis and the extent to which it exists in individuals largely determines their risk of having a heart attack.

CHD is a complex phenomenon that cannot always be clearly explained, and while we often do not know why some persons will suffer a heart attack and others not, studies have identified a number of factors that are associated with the incidence of CHD. These are often referred to as *CHD risk factors.*

THE RISK FACTORS

The most commonly accepted risk factors for CHD include: (1) smoking; (2) high blood pressure; (3) blood fat abnormalities (high cholesterol and low high-density lipoproteins); (4) age and sex; (5) family history; (6) diabetes; (7) lack of exercise; (8) stress; and (9) obesity.

Risk factors such as heredity, age, and sex cannot be controlled by the individual, but factors such as smoking, cholesterol, weight, high blood pressure, stress, and exercise can.

Cholesterol

The issue of the relationship of diet to CHD has been debated for decades. In a recent report issued by the National Cholesterol Education Program, endorsed by a coalition of thirty-eight federal agencies, and supported by such groups as the American Medical Association and the American Heart Association, it was recommended that all Americans over age 2 reduce the fat and cholesterol content of their diets in order to lower their risk of heart disease.

---

nation—even after the chest X rays have been viewed by an experienced radiologist—additional testing, such as an electrocardiogram or echocardiogram, may be necessary.

Elevated levels of cholesterol and fats in the blood have been associated with an increased risk of CHD, but the relationships are complex (see box "Cholesterol and Coronary Heart Disease"). Current recommendations are that the total daily fat content of the food we eat should be reduced from what is now 36 to 37 percent to an average of 30 percent or less of total calorie intake.

Weight

Obesity, often referred to as overweight but more accurately characterized as overfat, is a risk factor that is often accompanied by hypertension and a sedentary lifestyle. When a person loses weight and body fat, cholesterol and blood pressure levels are usually reduced. As is pointed out throughout this book, a well-designed CRE program can be most effective in losing weight and body fat.

Hypertension

Hypertension, or high blood pressure, is the most common disease of the circulatory system. Hypertension is diagnosed through blood pressure readings of the forces involved when the heart pumps blood through the arteries. Pressure is highest when the heart contracts to squeeze the blood into the arteries. This phase is referred to as the systolic pressure, with normal readings ranging from 120 to 140, as measured in millimeters of mercury recorded on an instrument called a sphygmomanometer. Systolic pressure tends to increase with age. Pressure is lowest as the heart relaxes and pressure on the artery walls eases. This is referred to as the diastolic pressure, with normal readings at 90 or less.

The causes of hypertension are varied and not completely clear. We know that it can develop in response to the hardening and narrowing of the arteries. Although there is no cure, hypertension can be controlled through weight reduction, medication, diet, and exercise. A report in April of 1990 in the British medical journal *Lancet* noted that for every 5 or 6 points that a person's blood pressure is reduced, the risk of heart attack declines by 20 to 25 percent. This analysis, which combines data from 37,000 people who participated in fourteen studies, concludes that benefits of lowering blood pressure result even for persons with only modestly elevated pressure.

People with hypertension may expect some improvement in resting blood pressure measurements as a result of CRE training. During active exercise, everyone's blood pressure, nonhypertensives and hypertensives alike, temporarily goes up because of more forceful and rapid heart contractions—a normal response to exercise. After activity is over, blood pressure returns to resting levels. Those with a higher CRE fitness level take less time for their pressure to return to normal. It also appears that both systolic and diastolic blood pressure levels can be lowered by a regular CRE exercise program. Regular programs of physical activity, in addition to drug therapy, are increasingly being prescribed to manage hypertension.

Smoking

Smokers face an increased risk of death as a result of CHD than nonsmokers. The more one smokes, and the stronger the cigarette, the greater the risk. Although smoking acts independently of other risk factors, when combined with high cholesterol and hypertension, the risk is sharply increased.

Stress

The amount of stress that one experiences every day and its relationship to CHD has been a controversial issue for many years. While we know that emotional stress can speed up the activity of the cardiovascular system and raise blood pressure, it is not altogether clear whether it is sustained stress and tension or being a particular personality type that can result in any permanent damage to the cardiovascular system.

Exercise

Physical inactivity, particularly a lack of aerobic exercise, has been associated with an increased risk of CHD. However, there are a number of other CRE training effects that deserve special attention because of their impact on the cardiovascular system.

CRE training may also reduce some people's blood cholesterol levels. High cholesterol levels have been found to be associated with an increased risk of coronary heart disease. (The evidence relating this to increased blood triglycerides, another body fat, is not nearly as convincing.) Recent research has shown that the relationship between cholesterol and exercise is more complex than once thought. The portion of blood cholesterol associated with high-density lipoproteins (HDL) actually is protective against coronary heart disease, while the opposite is true of low-density lipoproteins. Levels of HDL cholesterol have been found to be higher in people who regularly do CRE exercises than in those who don't.

It also has been shown that the blood of well-trained individuals has a decreased tendency to clot, thereby theoretically diminishing the possibility of heart attack. The exact role of exercise in preventing coronary heart disease, however, is not clear. Various population studies suggest that there are fewer heart attacks and sudden deaths from heart attack among physically active people than sedentary people. But it is difficult to tell whether active people live longer because their activity makes them healthier, or whether they live longer and are more active because they are healthier to begin with. None of the studies is conclusive, although some of them—including the renowned Framingham study, which has followed almost the entire community of Framingham, Massachusetts, for more than thirty years—have identified the risk factors mentioned above.

For these reasons, then, some authorities are convinced that exercises such as the model programs for CRE described in Chapter 7 can help to avert coronary heart disease and help to rehabilitate heart attack victims.

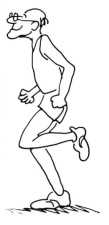

WHEN A HEART ATTACK OCCURS

As the arteries continue to narrow, less blood can flow through them to nourish the heart muscle. When the coronary arteries can no longer supply the heart muscle

Do active people live longer because of their activity or are they healthier to begin with?

CHOLESTEROL AND CORONARY HEART DISEASE

Cholesterol is a waxy substance (not a fat) manufactured by the body and essential to the performance of certain body functions. Cholesterol is carried in the blood where it is connected to large protein molecules called lipoproteins. There are several types of cholesterol-carrying lipoproteins, each with a different effect on the risk of CHD. They are low-density lipoproteins (LDL), which can cause clogging of the lining of the arteries and lead to heart disease; very low-density lipoproteins, which have also been implicated in the development of coronary heart disease; and high-density lipoproteins (HDL), which seem to protect against CHD by removing the cholesterol from the blood vessel walls and transporting it to the liver for disposal. In this connection LDL is often referred to as the "bad" and HDL as the "good" cholesterol.

Because of the different types of cholesterol, it can be confusing to interpret the various measures of cholesterol levels as they relate to the risk of heart disease. The first report of the National Cholesterol Education Program discusses risk in terms of total blood (serum) cholesterol levels as well as LDL and HDL levels. The report indicates that the "desirable" total cholesterol level for adults is less than 180 milligrams (per deciliter of blood). 200 milligrams is considered "borderline high," and levels of more than 240 milligrams represent "high risk." When using LDL levels alone, readings above 160 milligrams constitute "high risk," while levels of 130 to 159 are "borderline high."*

Many authorities believe that it is important to also consider HDL levels in order to get a better idea of coronary risk. In the case of HDL the higher the level, the better. Levels below 35 milligrams (higher for premenopausal women) may indicate high risk, even when the total cholesterol reading is normal.

Foods that contain particularly large quantities of cholesterol include egg yolks (not the whites), whole milk products, and meats. These foods are also rich in saturated fats, which can raise cholesterol levels.

One of the problems in reducing serum cholesterol is that rich sources of cholesterol and saturated fats also include some of the best sources of necessary fatty acids and complete proteins. Alternatives to the use of saturated fats are unsaturated fats. These include monounsaturated and polyunsaturated fats found in vegetable oils such as corn, safflower, cottonseed, soybean, sesame, sunflower, and olive. Monounsaturated and polyunsaturated fats tend to reduce total blood cholesterol and LDL levels. HDL levels can be increased by vigorous endurance exercise training and are difficult to raise by dietary means alone.

*The Consumers Union medical consultants accept less than 200 mg. as a desirable total cholesterol level, 200–240 mg. as "borderline high," and more than 260 as "high risk."

with oxygen, that portion of the heart nourished by the affected arteries dies (a condition known as myocardial infarction). If the area of heart muscle affected is not large, death from myocardial infarction may be prevented.

George is typical of a growing number of coronary heart disease victims whose recovery has been helped by exercise. Eight years earlier, because of severe chest pains, George had tests that showed there was blockage of a coronary artery. Given a choice between a coronary bypass operation and an exercise program to try to reduce the demands on his heart and improve his body's metabolic capacity, George chose exercise. In the beginning, he was in such poor shape that he had chest pain

Current recommendations call for our daily intake of cholesterol to be reduced to less than 300 milligrams a day. In addition, it is recommended that the total fat consumption of Americans be reduced from the current average of 36 to 37 percent of their daily calorie intake to an average of less than 30 percent, with saturated fats eliminated completely and the remainder of the daily fat intake derived from polyunsaturated and monounsaturated fats.

The Cardiovascular Disease Risk Chart for Cholesterol and Lipid Levels

Lipids	Age (yrs)	Excellent Protection 25th percentile (no changes necessary)		Moderate Risk 50th percentile (design your diet and exercise program from this text)		High Risk 75th percentile (consult physician for diet and/or drug therapy)		Very High Risk 90th percentile (seek immediate medical attention)	
		M	F	M	F	M	F*	M	F
Total	20–39	162–179	157–176	180–202	177–197	203–225	198–220	>225	>220
cholesterol	40–59	186–209	186–209	210–233	210–235	234–257	236–259	>257	>259
mg/dl	60+	189–213	205–227	214–240	228–252	241–262	253–276	>262	>276
LDL	20–39	100–117	90–108	118–137	109–127	138–159	128–149	>159	>149
cholesterol	40–59	119–140	110–128	141–162	129–155	163–183	156–181	>183	>181
mg/dl	60+	122–143	126–149	144–165	150–175	166–190	176–198	>190	>198
HDL	20–39	>51	>63	51–37	63–45	<37	<45 *	—	—
cholesterol	40–59	>52	>69	52–37	69–49	<37	<49	—	—
mg/dl	60+	>60	>74	60–40	74–50	<40	<50	—	—
Triglycerides	20–39	71–93	58–77	94–133	78–106	134–195	107–146 **	>195	>146
mg/dl	40–59	89–121	73–98	122–170	99–140	171–231	141–190	>231	>190
	60+	83–110	82–110	111–154	111–146	155–206	147–206	>206	>206
Total	20–39	2.3–3.6	1.9–2.8	3.7–5.1	2.9–3.6	5.2–6.1	3.7–4.2	>6.1	>4.2
cholesterol/	40–59	2.6–4.2	2.0–3.0	4.3–6.0	3.1–4.0	6.1–7.4	4.1–4.9	>7.4	>4.9
HDL ratio	60+	2.5–4.0	2.0–3.2	4.1–6.0	3.3–4.8	6.1–6.9	4.9–5.5	>6.9	>5.5

M = Male
F = Female

> = "more than"
< = "less than"

*Due to the lack of data, one may question whether HDL cholesterol levels in women in this range truly mean high risk. However, at this time, this is the best estimate of risk.

**Triglycerides at this level do not warrant drug therapy. Consult your physician/nutritionist for dietary, weight loss, or exercise therapy.

SOURCE: Kenneth Cooper, *Controlling Cholesterol* (New York: Bantam Books, 1988), p. 53.

with the slightest exertion. He started a regimen that included prescribed coronary medication and a carefully controlled program of exercise on a stationary bicycle. His progress was slow but steady: After seven years he had improved enough to begin a jogging program. Again he began slowly and modestly, with half-mile outings that included two or three walking intervals. A year later he was regularly jogging twenty miles a week, without any walking breaks, and he hoped soon to be doing four six-mile runs a week. His cardiologist finds his progress "unbelievable," and George agrees: "I'm in better physical condition than the average person without a cardiac problem who is not a regular exerciser."

George is an unusual example. Still, most cardiologists now recommend a gradual increase in exercise for people recovering from a heart attack or from heart surgery, and for people who may be at risk of heart attack. Such exercise programs must be approved by a physician and are usually carried out in a well-supervised facility.

CAN CORONARY HEART DISEASE BE REVERSED?

A topic subject to considerable debate and study is whether coronary artery disease can be reversed. More recent studies using diet and medication showed that it might be possible to slow down the process. New techniques that allow precise measurements of coronary artery diameters have made evaluation easier. One study has actually shown that the atherosclerotic process may even be reversible with diet. Such encouraging studies are few, but the word is out that diet is important.

SUDDEN CARDIAC DEATH IN YOUNG PEOPLE

Almost every year a story hits the news media about a young, fit athlete dying suddenly on the playing field. Although some of these deaths are due to coronary artery disease, most are due to congenital cardiac anomalies. Congenital cardiac anomalies are abnormal heart conditions present at birth. These conditions include an abnormal location of the coronary arteries, hypertrophic cardiomyopathy (enlarged and weakened heart muscle), and aortic stenosis (narrowing of the aorta, the large artery that delivers blood from the left ventricle of the heart).

Diseases of the heart valves are also a cause of sudden cardiac death in young people. Heart valve diseases can be present at birth, but they can also be caused by childhood diseases, such as rheumatic fever.

The good news is that exercise-related sudden death in young people is extremely rare. The bad news is that determining your risk is difficult and relatively expensive. Most of the contributing disorders are hard to detect during normal medical examinations. Probably the best screening technique is family history. If you have a family history of congenital heart disease or premature death from heart disease, see your doctor.

Some of these problems can now be controlled. For example, physicians have had great success in controlling high cholesterol, high blood pressure, and diabetes that runs in families. Individuals who previously would have been doomed to premature death are living normal lives thanks to new drugs and lifestyle modifications.

BEGINNING A CRE EXERCISE PROGRAM

If your self-assessment leads you to try to improve your CRE, you will need an exercise program designed specifically to help you meet that goal. To succeed with the program, however, will mean applying the two basic principles of fitness training—specificity and progressive overload.

Specificity

The training principle of specificity can help you narrow your choice to the activities best suited for improvement of CRE. These are the ones that use large muscle groups steadily and rhythmically—activities such as walking, jogging, swimming, bicycling, cross-country skiing, rope skipping, and hiking. All of these are effective because they require large amounts of energy, thus burning a large number of calories. (This makes many of these same activities well suited for reducing body fat or losing weight.) Keeping track of the number of calories burned in a particular exercise program is a convenient way to measure the energy requirement of the activity. The greater the amount of energy expended, the greater the amount of oxygen that your cardiorespiratory system will deliver to the muscles.

Activities effective for CRE are self-paced—you can control progressive overload by adjusting the intensity, duration, and frequency of your exercise sessions as your fitness increases. Such adjustments may be more difficult with competitive sports. If you choose tennis or basketball as your CRE exercise, for example, the intensity of your play may not be within your control. Your skills may be so minimal that you won't be active enough to get a training effect. Or you may get discouraged or bored if your level of skills is better or worse than those of the competition. Or in the excitement of the game, you may push yourself beyond a comfortable level of intensity. As noted, aerobic activities are those that rhythmically use the large muscle groups such as those in the legs.

Progressive Overload

No matter which specific activity you choose, you will need to base your exercise program on the principle of progressive overload. The idea is to begin with your current exercise level and gradually expose your body to increasing demands. The way you achieve overload will depend on which combinations of intensity, duration, and frequency of workout suits you best. In a twenty-week study comparing walking and jogging, for example, one group of men participated in fast walking for forty minutes, four days a week while another group jogged for thirty minutes, three days a week. The higher intensity of the jogging program was offset by the increased duration and frequency of the walking program, so that both groups expended the same total amount of energy each week. The amount of overload—and the extent of CRE improvement—was the same in both groups.

So if you stick to proper combinations of intensity, duration, and frequency, you can improve CRE whether you walk, jog, swim, cycle, ski, skip rope, or hike. Even though these activities demand different levels of exertion, thus burning different numbers of calories per minute, all can produce CRE training effects. Choose the one that most appeals to you and that you can expect to practice regularly all year round. (Keep in mind that although jogging three miles in thirty minutes every other day may be sufficient if you wish to improve and maintain general cardiorespiratory fitness, such a regimen would not make you a competitive runner.)

Intensity

You won't get CRE training effects unless the intensity of your workout is high enough to raise your heart rate sufficiently above its usual resting level and to keep it there for at least twenty minutes. You need not raise your heart rate to its maximum rate to get CRE improvement, however. Just keep your heart rate higher than its resting rate and lower than its maximum rate—within what we call the exercise benefit zone (EBZ). Your maximum heart rate (MHR) and EBZ can both be established fairly simply by following the procedures outlined below.

MHR and EBZ   If you have had a cardiac stress test that took your heart rate to maximum, the test facility can probably tell you your precise maximum heart rate per minute—the heart rate you achieved at maximum intensity during the test period. Stress test data are not essential, however. You can estimate your maximum heart rate very easily by subtracting your age from the figure 220. If you are 20 years old, then, your estimated maximum heart rate is 200.

Finding your exercise benefit zone—between 70 and 85 percent of maximum heart rate—is almost as simple. All you have to do is make two calculations, based on the MHR, to establish your EBZ.* Once you have a maximum heart rate—either exact or estimated—just multiply it by .70 to find the lower threshold of your EBZ and by .85 to find the upper limit. Figure 3-1 shows estimated MHRs and EBZs for ages 15 through 75. For example, if you are 20 years old, your estimated MHR is 200 and your EBZ is between 140 and 170. To achieve CRE training effects when you exercise, you would need to maintain your heart rate within your EBZ for twenty minutes or more per exercise session.

Remember, you should not exercise at maximum heart rate to achieve training effects. Training at near maximum heart rate on a regular basis increases the risk of muscle and joint injury. As long as you raise your heart rate into the EBZ, you will

---

*The American College of Sports Medicine recommends, and many people use, a procedure known as the Karvonen method to calculate the EBZ. The Karvonen method considers the EBZ as between 60 and 90 percent of *maximum heart rate reserve:* Maximum heart rate minus resting heart rate multiplied by .60 plus resting heart rate equals 60 percent of heart rate reserve. We prefer a simpler calculation that places the EBZ between 70 and 85 percent of MHR, with the resting heart rate not included in the computation.

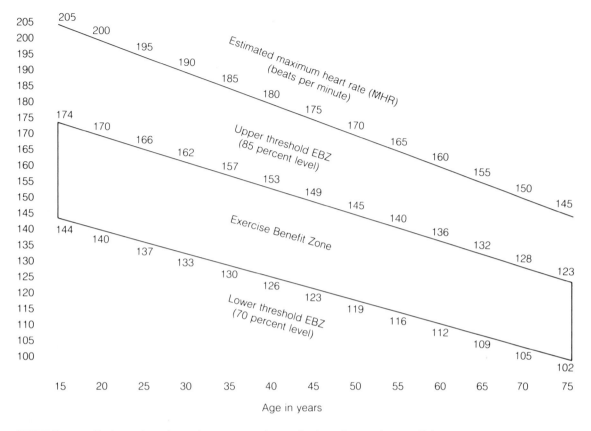

FIGURE 3-1   Estimated maximum heart rate and exercise benefit zone by age. Subtract your age from 220 to get your estimated maximum heart rate (MHR). Find that figure on the top line. Below that figure you can find the upper threshold and the lower threshold of your EBZ. Example: If you are 20 years old, your estimated MHR is 200 (220 − 20), and your EBZ thresholds are 170 (upper) and 140 (lower).

make progress. Within that range of intensity, you can vary the amount of your over-load at will. The magnitude of training effects increases with the extent of the over-load, but you can keep intensity relatively low and still get training effects by overloading duration or frequency.

All you must do to achieve improvement in CRE is to maintain your heart rate within your EBZ for at least twenty minutes during your regular exercise sessions. It is not necessary to raise your heart rate to higher and higher levels. Just stay in your EBZ. For example, Ray, an 18-year-old, told us that he regularly runs a five-mile course with a heart rate of 140 beats per minute. When he established this routine, he was running the course in about fifty minutes. Some months later his time had dropped to forty minutes, and a month after that it was down to thirty-eight minutes. Both distance and heart rate remained the same, but Ray's increase in CRE let him increase the speed of his run, thus shortening the duration of his exercise period.

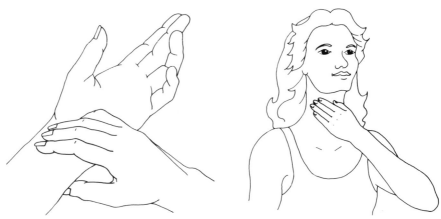

FIGURE 3-2   Taking radial (left) and carotid (right) pulse.

Taking Your Pulse   To be sure that you are exercising hard enough to keep your heart rate within your EBZ, you may have to learn how to take your pulse.* You can do this using either the radial artery or the carotid artery (Figure 3-2); both are near enough to the skin for you to feel them easily. To locate the radial artery, place the tips of the middle three fingers of your right hand on the left wrist in the little groove below the base of your left thumb. To locate the carotid artery, place the tips of the three middle fingers of one hand on your neck under the jaw bone, about midway between the chin and the ear. Hold your fingertips on one of these points with sufficient pressure to feel the artery pulsating—each pulsation reflecting a heartbeat. Avoid excessive pressure on the carotid artery. Using a stopwatch (push the start button and begin counting) or a watch with a sweep-second hand, count the number of pulse beats in ten seconds. To determine your heart rate per minute, multiply by 6.

You can use Table 3-1 to compute your EBZ in terms of your 10-second pulse rate. That can save you the trouble of having to multiply in the midst of a workout. Start counting your pulse immediately after exercising because the heart rate drops significantly within fifteen seconds. By stopping your exercise briefly and taking your pulse right away, you can readily determine whether your exercise is keeping your heart rate within your EBZ.

If you don't want to interrupt your exercise to take your pulse, try the "talk test": You are probably at the lower end of your EBZ if you can comfortably hold a

---

*The January 1980 issue of *Consumer Reports* discussed a number of automated pulse recorders. These gadgets could help people under close medical supervision, but Consumers Union's medical consultants thought they were cumbersome and expensive. The February 1980 issue of *Consumer Reports* discussed a heart rate monitor that not only recorded your pulse but let you program the upper and lower heart rate limits that define your EBZ. An alarm sounded when your pulse was outside your EBZ. This equipment had its flaws (erratic readings, rather complex program sequences, and the like) and was expensive. But it might be worth the investment if you find such equipment motivating.

TABLE 3-1   Exercise Benefit Zones for Various Ages

To improve CRE, an exercise should bring your heart rate to your exercise benefit zone (EBZ)—between 70 and 85 percent of your maximum heart rate (MHR)—and should maintain your heart rate within your EBZ. The table provides estimated MHR per minute and the EBZ for various ages. The table also gives you the number of beats per minute at the 70 percent and 85 percent levels of EBZ.

| | | Exercise Benefit Zone | | | |
| | | 70% estimated MHR | | 85% estimated MHR | |
Age	Estimated MHR per minute	60 sec.	10 sec.	60 sec.	10 sec.
15	205	144	24	174	29
20	200	140	23	170	28
25	195	137	23	166	28
30	190	133	22	162	27
35	185	130	22	157	26
40	180	126	21	153	26
45	175	123	21	149	25
50	170	119	20	145	24
55	165	116	19	140	24
60	160	112	19	136	23
65	155	109	18	132	22
70	150	105	18	128	21
75	145	102	17	123	21

conversation while exercising. With experience, some people can learn to judge whether they are in the EBZ without stopping to check their pulse.

The EBZ is, at best, an approximation. (See Table 3-1 for approximate EBZs for different age groups.) It is important for you to monitor how your body feels on any particular day. "Listen" to your body. You may have to increase or reduce your exercise intensity to adapt to a variety of circumstances. Your reaction to exercise may vary in response to such environmental factors as temperature, humidity, or altitude, and to such personal variables as infection, medication, fatigue, and psychological stress.

Duration

The duration of an exercise period will depend, of course, on how strenuous the exercise is. In general, the harder you work, the shorter the time you must spend to achieve the desired effect. But if you are exercising at high intensity near the upper limit of your EBZ, you may exhaust yourself quickly. If you are exercising close to the lower threshold of your EBZ, you will be able to continue longer.

There is some evidence that you can get a training effect by working at or above the upper limit of your EBZ for as little as five or ten minutes. But because the potential for injury—especially among beginners—is greater with more strenuous exercise, the likelihood of continued improvement is lower. We recommend that a CRE exercise period should last at least fifteen minutes (not including warm-up or

YOUR FITNESS PROFILE 3-1
Computing Your Exercise Benefit Zone

Objective: To determine your exercise benefit zone.

Directions: Compute your predicted maximum heart rate per minute (HRM) by subtracting your age from 220. Then multiply your estimated HRM by .70 and .85. The result is called the exercise benefit zone (EBZ). Because during exercise you will count your own pulse rate for just 10 seconds, it is helpful to know your minimum and maximum "10-second conversion" EBZs. To compute it, divide your minimum and maximum EBZs by 6.

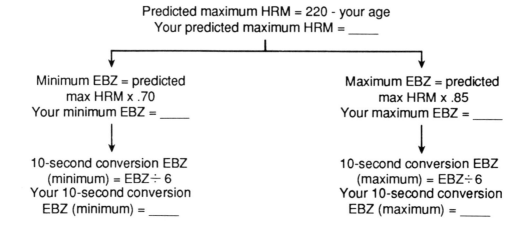

Predicted maximum HRM = 220 - your age
Your predicted maximum HRM = _____

Minimum EBZ = predicted
max HRM x .70
Your minimum EBZ = _____

10-second conversion EBZ
(minimum) = EBZ ÷ 6
Your 10-second conversion
EBZ (minimum) = _____

Maximum EBZ = predicted
max HRM x .85
Your maximum EBZ = _____

10-second conversion EBZ
(maximum) = EBZ ÷ 6
Your 10-second conversion
EBZ (maximum) = _____

cool-down). For an exerciser to sustain an activity for the minimum twenty minutes may mean having to work at the lower end of the EBZ. Our experience with thousands of York College students age 18 to over 70 suggests that at the beginning of an exercise program your activity period should last at least twenty minutes and that, as you become adjusted to the work load, you should add increased time at a rate of no more than 10 percent a week.

Beginners should progress very gradually to greater durations and higher intensities. Studies with joggers indicate that low-intensity exercise for long durations helps avoid injuries and minimize discomfort. At least eight or ten weeks of slowly increasing the duration of training may be necessary for most beginners. It may even be advisable to start at an intensity considerably below your EBZ until your muscles adjust to the demands of your program. As you increase the intensity of the workout, and as the training effects begin to accrue, you may find yourself increasing the duration of your exercise sessions simply because they have become an enjoyable experience.

Nancy told Consumers Union that when she first took up running she could barely finish a quarter mile. She found it boring and mindless but persisted because she felt it was "doing her a lot of good." After a year of training, her endurance had increased until she could cover six miles regularly in sixty-three minutes. She slept "amazingly well" and could eat "practically anything without putting on weight." At that point, she bought her second pair of running shoes, joined a local running club, and admitted that somewhere between three miles and five miles, she had actually begun to enjoy it.

The higher the intensity or the longer the duration of the exercise session (or possibly both, as you get used to the activity), the greater will be the improvement in your CRE. A little experimentation with the structure of your exercise regimen will help you find the best way to adjust intensity and duration to get maximum improvement in CRE. The combinations are almost infinite. You can always vary them to suit your particular needs and interests and adjust them regularly to relieve boredom and maintain motivation.

Frequency

Frequency of exercise, for the beginner, need not be more than three or four days a week for most activities. In fact, jogging and running more frequently than that may increase the chance of injury, particularly for the beginner. Three days a week, or about every other day, is adequate to achieve improvement in CRE. (Athletes usually require more training time.)

Some people, however, don't like to skip a day between exercising. If you prefer a routine of, say, six days a week, feel rested enough before each workout, and have no muscular or joint problems (as is often reported by overzealous joggers), the almost daily routine may help to develop even higher levels of CRE. Such a schedule would certainly be useful if you also wanted to achieve and maintain lean body composition. If you want to exercise more than every other day, it might be wise to alternate the type of CRE exercise you do, especially if you are prone to injury and want to avoid muscular or joint problems. For example, you might run one day and swim the next, or you might alternate bicycling one day with taking a brisk walk the next.

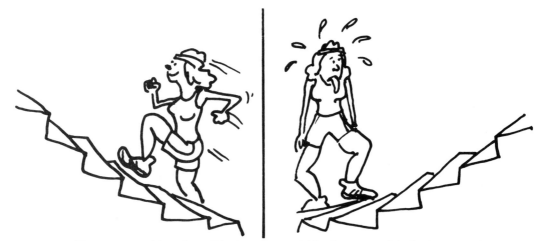

If you stop exercising, deconditioning occurs quickly; the same activity begins to require more effort.

It's important to continue exercising. When you are inactive, deconditioning occurs fairly quickly. A study from the Universities of Maryland and Kentucky reported on a group of women who exercised for ten weeks and made significant gains in CRE. When they later dropped their training for five weeks, they lost almost 70 percent of their CRE gains. After ten weeks without exercise, they were back where they had started before the training program began. In another study, conducted by investigators at Wake Forest University, a group of men jogged eight miles a week for twenty weeks. Twelve weeks later, those who had dropped down to less than five miles a week had lost about 50 percent of their gains. Those who kept to a routine of about eight miles a week continued to improve in CRE.

These studies confirm our belief that a workout within the EBZ about every other day is necessary to maintain cardiorespiratory fitness. Less frequent exercise will not only fall short of producing training effects, it may also allow deconditioning to occur.

CALORIES AS A MEASURE OF CRE EXERCISE

The amount of work you do in the exercise regimen you select depends on how you adjust and combine intensity, duration, and frequency to achieve progressive overload. One measure of that work is the energy you expend in doing it. And the simplest way to keep track of energy is by noting the number of calories you burn. If the activity you choose meets the basic principles of specificity and progressive overload, and if you know the total calories you burn in that activity, you can judge whether your exercise regimen is appropriate for achieving CRE training effects.

As we will see in Chapter 4, the calorie is a unit of heat. It's commonly used to indicate not only the potential energy in food, but also the energy expended to perform work. By adjusting intensity, duration, and frequency in various combinations, you can raise or lower the total number of calories you expend in your exercise sessions.

Table 3-2 illustrates how you can use varied combinations of duration and frequency to achieve CRE goals. The CRE potential of an activity depends on its ability to bring the heart rate into the EBZ. An activity that keeps your heart rate at the low end of the EBZ is a low-intensity activity. And one that raises your heart rate to the upper limits is a high-intensity activity.

If you choose an activity that burns more calories per minute than another activity—a high-intensity activity, for example, such as running instead of walking—you might be able to shorten the amount of time you need to spend on your exercise sessions to achieve your CRE goal. Or you could perform a high-intensity exercise at the top range of your EBZ: You could run at 85 percent of your maximum heart rate, which would burn more calories per minute than running at 70 percent.

But a high-intensity exercise won't necessarily improve CRE more than a low-intensity one (or exercising at the low end of your EBZ). In fact, exercise done at lower intensity may burn more calories overall because it can usually be continued for longer periods at reduced intensity. For instance, pedaling your bike uphill is a high-intensity activity burning many more calories per minute than pedaling at the same speed on a level road. But you can keep up the low-intensity pedaling on the level road longer and thus burn more calories in a single session than in the brief but more intense uphill effort.

Some authorities believe a minimum number of calories must be expended if exercise is to provide protection against heart attack. A retrospective study by Ralph S. Paffenbarger, Jr., a professor of epidemiology at Stanford University, showed that Harvard alumni who burned 2,000 or more calories a week through

---

TABLE 3-2   Calorie Guide to CRE

The table shows how you can adjust duration and frequency when exercising within your EBZ to establish the number of calories you need to burn per week to attain your CRE goals.

Calories used per week	Duration (minutes per session)	Frequency (days per week)	CRE level
250–500	15–20	3–4	Primarily for beginners with low CRE.
501–750	15–30	3–4	For those who wish to progress from low to moderate levels of CRE.
751–1,250	31–45	3–4	For those who wish to progress from moderate to high levels of CRE.
1,251–2,000	31–45	4–6	To achieve and maintain a very high level of CRE.
Over 2,000	31–60	4–6	To achieve and maintain a very high level of CRE; to try for possible heart-disease prevention benefits.

exercise had fewer heart attacks than those who got less exercise. (Interestingly enough, Paffenbarger found that former varsity athletes who did not maintain a high level of activity after graduation were more at risk than those who had been non-athletes in their student days but who later became physically active.) Thomas Cureton, another authority on fitness, has suggested that burning 300 calories a session is helpful.

You may wish to undertake a CRE program using a calorie goal. If so, choose an exercise regimen that has the potential of relatively high caloric expenditure yet would permit you to reduce or increase intensity, duration, and frequency as your fitness level directs.

EXERCISE SYSTEMS AND CRE

You can make a good deal of progress on a well-planned CRE program suited to your interests and abilities. Your progress, however, can be affected by the exercise system you choose to follow. Many people who exercise for CRE use a *continuous rhythmic technique* (CRT), which involves jogging, cycling, or swimming at a set pace for a set time. This system has simplicity as its chief advantage: Once you calculate your EBZ, all you have to do is choose a pace that will maintain your heart rate within the EBZ for the duration of your workout. CRT involves a relatively slow pace, continued for long distances. As CRE improves, the pace gets picked up automatically. CRT practitioners seem to enjoy the system because its simplicity allows for a period of pure activity, a time when few decisions have to be made and the body can proceed "on automatic."

For beginners, CRT can have some disadvantages. Because of low CRE, they may become fatigued and fail to last through an exercise session. Or the simplicity of the format and the monotony of the pace may become boring, tempting them to give up.

One way to get around the negative effects of a program based on CRT is to interrupt the exercise with *interval training*. This system shortens the periods of high-intensity activity by introducing brief periods of rest or low-intensity activity. Interval training allows your body to recuperate partially from the high-intensity work, permitting you to complete a longer total period of work without becoming exhausted or bored. These intervals of high- and low-intensity activity can be repeated until you have finished the number of sets you planned to do.

Here's how interval training works. Suppose twenty minutes is your best time for jogging two miles while maintaining your heart rate within your EBZ. And suppose your rate of speed is six miles per hour (ten minutes per mile). With interval training, you can run one-half mile in five minutes (or even slightly faster), followed by a one-eighth-mile walk at three miles per hour. If you alternate these four times, your total distance will be two and one-half miles. The exercise duration will then become thirty minutes instead of the twenty minutes that was your manageable limit with continuous rhythmic activity. And you will have burned approximately 280 calories instead of 250. Naturally, the exact number of calories you burn depends on your weight.

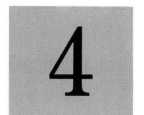

Body Composition

After you've read this chapter, you will be able to:

Differentiate between *overweight, overfat,* and *obesity.*

Recognize how calorie balance affects the gain or loss of body fat.

Identify the limitations of crash diets for reducing body fat.

Recognize the elements of an effective exercise program for controlling body fat.

Identify common myths connected with efforts to change body composition.

"In my lifetime I suppose I have lost approximately five hundred pounds!" So began a letter from Gwen, a 45-year-old. Like many other people, she undertook a physical fitness program primarily to lose weight.

Others told us they wanted to firm up or slim down. For many, the decision to lose weight or to shed fat had a tone of determination. "At age thirty-two," reported Jesse, describing his moment of truth, "I stood nude before a full-length mirror and, frowning with disgust, realized that my chest had slid down into my belly." He still weighed the same 200 pounds he had as a 17-year-old football player, but his waist was now 40 inches. Lesley, a 26-year-old, had a similar confrontation. "I finally couldn't pretend any more," she confessed. "When I looked in the mirror, I could see it. . . . I decided it had to stop there."

For some people, the turning point came in their doctor's office. Sixty-six-year-old Darren discovered some years ago that he had a tendency toward diabetes. Following his doctor's advice, he took off fifteen pounds with the aid of a stationary bicycle and calisthenics. "Thanks to the loss of weight and the increase in the amount of exercise," wrote Darren, "I have been able to control my blood sugar without drugs." Ironically, Darren had begun his forty-year commitment to exercise when he joined a "Y" to *gain* weight. After five years, he had progressed from 127 to 165 pounds and then worked to keep himself at that weight by exercising at least three times a week.

Most people, of course, want to lose weight. Rosa, a college senior, was upset to find that she weighed six pounds more than she did as an entering freshman. At 5 feet 5 inches tall and 130 pounds, she does not have excessive body fat, but, as is so often the case among women, she has unrealistic standards regarding leanness. We find that some women are more influenced by standards of leanness set by glamour magazines than by a more realistic understanding of nature's effects on a woman's body composition.

OVERWEIGHT, OVERFAT, AND OBESE

It's no surprise that physicians often figure so prominently in reports of weight loss. Although obesity is not a primary risk factor for coronary heart disease, it can be a danger signal, particularly in someone with one or more of the known risk factors. Loss of weight, especially when it's the side effect of a regular exercise program, may lessen the chance of coronary heart disease, speed rehabilitation after a heart attack, and prevent a recurrence. You can also reduce problems related to diabetes, gallbladder disease, and hypertension (high blood pressure) by weight loss.

Estimates vary, but there are probably 50 to 80 million Americans—up to half the adult and adolescent population—who are overweight. What this means in most cases is that these people weigh more than the so-called ideal weight for their height and build. Others may not be overweight by the charts but they feel—and look—overfat. In contrast, the charts may lump a few into the overweight category when their excess weight is actually due to muscle development rather than too much body fat.

If you've done the self-assessment tests in Chapter 1 to determine the proportion of body fat to muscle, you should know how you rate in terms of body composition. For men, more than 25 percent body fat indicates obesity; men whose body fat is between 20 and 25 percent are overfat. Women with more than 35 percent body fat are considered to be obese; with more than 30 percent, they are overfat.

The nature of obesity (and overfatness) can be mystifying. Not until the 1960s was there a breakthrough in understanding obesity. It was then that Jules Hirsch and his colleagues at Rockefeller University in New York City showed that fat people have extra-large fat cells and, interestingly, that they have more fat cells than thinner people. When a fat person loses weight on a low-calorie diet, it is the size of each fat cell that decreases, not the number of fat cells, except in the grossly obese person. The number of fat cells probably remains constant from about adolescence onward.

Because of the significance of the childhood years in the development of fat cells, people concerned about children's health should—after consultation with a physician—encourage calorie restriction when appropriate. And they should encourage regular, vigorous exercise for children. Obesity can never be cured. It can be controlled, however, by maintaining a balance between eating (the amount of calories ingested) and physical activity (the amount of calories burned). If young children and teenagers are encouraged to shun excess calories and to exercise regularly, they can minimize the problem of obesity in adulthood.

If you were unable to assess your body composition by using any of the methods described in Chapter 1, you may be able to make a rough judgment on the basis of more casual evidence. Has your weight gone up continually over the years? If so, the additional weight has probably been in the form of fat. You may be a victim of "creeping obesity," like Brian, a 28-year-old former college athlete, who weighed 145 at graduation but six sedentary years later weighs 175 pounds.

As Brian did, you may have been putting on weight slowly but steadily over a period of years. Even if you haven't gained an ounce since your teens, your activity level may have declined. If so, it is likely that some muscles may have decreased in size and some fat deposits may have increased in size. This process is inevitable with aging, but it proceeds at a slower rate in people who are physically active. As a result, you may decide that your goal is not so much weight reduction as fat reduction, or what many people call toning up the body—increasing muscular fitness and making muscles stronger.

CALORIES AND ENERGY

Whether your goal is to improve body composition or to reduce total weight, your approach will be the same: to lose fat. Almost always, steps taken to reduce body fat will also lower body weight. Theories and methods of weight control come and go, but most authorities now agree that weight control is best achieved by a combination of strategies calling for both a balanced diet and regular exercise. The positive effects on weight reduction of reduced dietary intake and increased exercise output are most readily illustrated in terms of calories.

Energy is measured in kilocalories, the amount of heat required to raise the temperature of one kilogram of water 1 degree (from 14.5 to 15.5 degrees centigrade). Kilocalories are commonly referred to as calories. Calories are used to measure the potential energy value of the food we eat and of the energy we expend in performing work. In an effort to standardize scientific language, the unit of measurement for energy is the joule. Although the joule is used in scientific papers, it has not yet received widespread acceptance by the public.

One pound of body fat is equal to roughly 3,500 calories. If the food you eat in a day supplies 3,500 calories and you burn 3,500 calories in doing the day's work, you are in *neutral calorie balance:* You will neither gain nor lose weight. If, however, the next day you have a lighter work schedule, and if you take in 4,000 calories and you burn only 2,300 calories, you will have a *positive calorie balance* of 1,700 calories. These 1,700 surplus calories—whether consumed as protein, carbohydrate, or fat—will show up eventually as about one-half pound of body fat, stored in fat cells, ready to be converted into a reserve supply of energy should the need arise. If no need arises, the fat deposits remain where they are.

If on the following day you resume your normal work load, expending 3,500 calories but taking in only 1,800 calories, you will be in *negative calorie balance* to the tune of 1,700 calories. Your body will have to call upon its reserve of fat for your energy needs that day. Theoretically, you would lose about one-half pound of fat. If you stay in positive calorie balance for a significant time by either eating more or exercising less, you will gain weight by adding fat to your body. If you stay in negative calorie balance for a prolonged period by either eating less or exercising more, you will lose weight by using up some of your fat reserve. If you stay in neutral calorie balance, using up all the calories you take in each day, your weight will not change. Theoretically, it's as simple as that.

As most of us know, however, it isn't that simple at all. Even a small regular increase in daily calorie intake can markedly affect your weight. Suppose you begin to consume 250 extra calories a day—say, two thick slices of bread and butter—without any change in your activity pattern. You could then count on gaining about a pound every two weeks. At the end of a year, you would have put on some twenty-six pounds—just from a mere 250 more calories a day. It would be a different story, of course, if you began a new exercise program or increased your activities when you increased your food intake. That way you could maintain a neutral calorie balance or even work for a negative calorie balance—and lose weight.

CRASH DIETS

Resist the temptation to begin your weight reduction campaign by going on a crash diet. Most of these so-called miracle cures for obesity require such drastic changes in your regular eating habits that you're not likely to stick with them for very long. And if you do maintain the diet, you could be compromising your health. Instead, we suggest you take a more conservative approach to weight loss. It requires more perseverance but offers a greater probability of success because it calls for less disruption of your customary eating patterns.

Most crash diets are based on ill-considered, half-understood, or pseudo-scientific theories. Some of these diets place a potentially dangerous emphasis on certain kinds of foods to the neglect or exclusion of others. Many fad diets rely on a drastic reduction in or even elimination of dietary carbohydrate. Cutting back on carbohydrate reduces the glycogen (stored carbohydrate) in muscles and liver. With every gram of lost carbohydrate, there is also a loss of about three grams of body water. The dramatic loss of five or more pounds almost immediately after you go on such a diet is almost entirely attributable to a sudden increase in urinary output. You have not lost any fat—just fluid. Fat cannot usually be lost that rapidly. And weight loss due to fluid loss is easily regained. What seemed like instant success could turn into a discouraging setback.

Lean body mass, or fat-free weight, accounts for about 40 percent of weight loss during the first two weeks of a crash diet. Lean body mass mainly consists of skeletal muscle. Amino acids (the building blocks of proteins) are used to make blood sugar in the liver during periods of starvation (the body perceives a crash diet as a period of starvation). If you think about people who have lost a lot of weight in a short time, they usually look like they have lost a lot of muscle mass. They don't look toned. That's because the crash diet resulted in the loss of lean body mass. The ideal diet helps you maintain lean body mass and body water and lose body fat. This is only accomplished by losing weight gradually, over a long period of time.

Moreover, if you increase your activity level to create a negative calorie balance, you will need a well-balanced diet. It would be imprudent, if not downright dangerous, to undertake an exercise program without meeting your nutritional needs. It would be much wiser to reduce your caloric intake slightly, being sure to include adequate protein, carbohydrate, fat, vitamins, and minerals. At the same time, increase your activity enough to ensure a negative calorie balance. With such a regimen, you should be able to lose weight slowly but steadily. Chapter 8 contains specific diet suggestions along with some exercise tips for controlling weight.

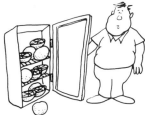

Single food diets can actually hurt more than help you.

EXERCISE AND DIET

We used to ask prospective physical education teachers in our classes whether they thought exercise had any part in weight reduction. The majority—at the beginning of the term, at any rate—ruled out exercise, insisting that only diet was important. They claimed it was impossible—or at least impractical—to lose weight through exercise. You would have to jog seven hours to burn the 3,500 calories needed to lose one pound, their argument went. Who could jog for seven hours? The fallacy, of course, is that you need not burn all 3,500 calories at one time, any more than you would necessarily take in the 3,500 calories all at one meal. Actually, if you jog only a half-hour a day, after fourteen days you will have completed seven hours of jogging. At the rate of 500 calories an hour, you would have established a negative calorie balance of 3,500 calories over those two weeks—provided, of course, that you maintained your normal calorie intake and carried on all your other activities as usual during those two weeks.

Losing one pound in two weeks may not seem like much, especially contrasted with the lure of a crash diet that promises a twenty-pound loss in the same time. But if you were to maintain prudent eating patterns and jog every day for a year, you would actually lose twenty-six pounds, six more than the crash diet tempted you with. And you would have a much better chance of keeping the weight off than if you had starved yourself for two weeks on a crash diet. If, in addition to jogging, you also decreased your caloric intake by as little as 250 calories a day (cutting out those two thick slices of bread and butter, for example), you would create an even greater negative calorie balance and so lose weight a bit more rapidly than by exercise alone.

Appetite and Exercise

People used to think that appetite invariably increases with exercise. That is usually not the case, especially with part-time exercisers who work out three to five days a week for a relatively brief time. Studies have shown that, over a period of months, most people who exercise strenuously for more than thirty minutes but less than one hour experience little if any change in appetite, and they succeed in losing weight.

An unusually heavy work load, however, does affect appetite. A construction worker who does six to seven hours of heavy muscular labor day in and day out or a dancer who spends six to seven hours a day in class, rehearsal, and performance may require a diet relatively high in calories to support their extremely high levels of activity. Similarly, the average person who spends a long vacation day on a ski trail or backpacking—and burns unaccustomed amounts of calories—will probably be ravenous at dinner. But this increase in appetite does not hold true for people who exercise regularly for shorter time spans. And even those who do get an increase in appetite—and therefore increase their food intake somewhat—still manage to lose weight as long as they are careful to remain in negative calorie balance.

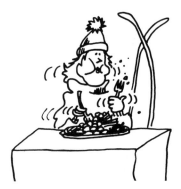

Shorter and regular exercise sessions do not prompt the increase in appetite that longer and sporadic workouts do.

Diet Without Exercise

If you want to improve your body composition as well as lose weight—that is, if your self-assessment has shown that you're not merely overweight but overfat—you probably want to increase your ratio of muscle to fat while you take off excess pounds. There is some evidence that dieting alone may cause you to lose muscle as well as fat. In one controlled study, for example, a group of twenty-five overweight women lost between 10.6 and 12 pounds in sixteen weeks. One subgroup of the women reduced their daily food intake by 500 calories. Another subgroup increased their daily activities to burn an additional 500 calories each. The remainder reduced their dietary intake by just 250 calories—maintaining the same percentage relationship among protein, carbohydrate, and fat—and stepped up their exercise to burn 250 additional calories. All three groups lost roughly the same amount of weight. But the diet-only group lost lean muscle tissue as well as body fat, while the exercise-only group and the diet-and-exercise group both gained in muscle rather than lost. What's more, they lost more fat than did the diet-only group.

CHOOSING A SENSIBLE REGIMEN

A reasonable goal for weight loss is no more than one pound a week. Over a year's time, even if you lost one-half pound a week, you'd be lighter by about twenty-six pounds. To lessen the chance of losing lean muscle tissue along with fat, you should increase your level of exercise as well as decrease calorie intake while accomplishing the weight loss.

Particularly important for changing body composition and for losing weight are the duration and frequency of your exercise program. (Intensity is less important for improvement in this fitness component.) For most people, a duration of thirty minutes and a frequency of at least three times a week seem to be the *minimum* requirements for altering body composition and achieving weight loss.

In one study, for example, women who were 10 to 60 percent overweight did not begin to lose weight until the duration of a walking program was more than thirty minutes a day. Over a year, the women—who were subject to no dietary restrictions—lost an average of twenty-two pounds each. In another study, thirty-minute sessions twice a week of a walking/jogging/running program were not enough to change body composition, while the same program four times a week did reduce body fat significantly.

Increasing duration and frequency can increase the rate of change. Consider Mick, who described his regimen of running about six miles in forty-five minutes almost every day. "When I started running," he wrote, "I was 160 pounds, 5 feet 9 inches. I knew that I burned 100 calories for every mile that I ran, so I expected to lose some weight. But I did not expect to now weigh about 135 pounds, a loss of twenty-five pounds!" Mick says he hadn't wanted to lose that much weight and even had increased his food intake by snacking. He now feels "fantastic at 135 pounds."

Which Exercise Is Best?

Cardiorespiratory endurance (CRE)—or aerobic—activities, such as walking, jogging, running, swimming, and bicycling, are the most useful for losing weight because they eventually burn more calories than do muscle-strengthening exercises, such as weight training or calisthenics. Weight training, however, can increase muscle tissue and thereby increase the proportion of muscle to fat. The sedentary and relatively inactive person may take comfort in the knowledge that walking is as effective for weight loss as bicycling or running, as long as you pay proper attention to duration and frequency of exercise. The overweight women in the walking program cited earlier walked for more than thirty minutes a day every day for a year and—with no dietary restrictions at all—lost from ten to thirty-eight pounds.

Remember that you can increase the total calories expended while performing an activity if you prolong duration even if you have to reduce intensity to do so. In other words, to change body composition you probably would be better off walking for an hour than jogging for twenty minutes. Calories do count, after all, but they count much more if you count them on the road as well as on the plate.

To decide which exercise to select as part of a body composition regimen, consult Profile 4-1, which lists a variety of fitness activities and the calories expended for each. (These activities are a sampling of those listed in Appendix B.)

A strategy for changing body composition need not be based exclusively on a formal exercise program, however. Practically any everyday activity uses up calories. Several *Consumer Reports* readers told us they had healthy appetites but maintained their weight by combining regular exercise with a vigorous approach to routine daily tasks. For example, Veronica, 19, runs from one part of the campus to another to attend classes. As far as she is concerned, this is part of her exercise routine. In fact, everything she does is potential exercise: "Even when I do housework, I try to do it in a brisk manner and not just clean."

Profiles 4-2 and 4-3 list nonsport and sedentary activities and their calorie costs. To determine the value of these nonsport activities for weight reduction, apply the same criteria as you would for any of the exercises or activities listed in Profile 4-1. Obviously, if you're going to rely on dressing, eating your meals, and writing letters to help you lose weight, you won't make much progress. Such activities use few calories per minute and don't usually last for long. However, if you chop wood or build a home-entertainment center, you're much more likely to experience weight loss. Such activities are more effective for weight loss than, say, getting dressed, because they expend more calories and require more of your time to do them. In fact, you're likely to burn calories at about the same rate as for many active sports. For even greater success in weight loss, supplement your exercise program—and your routine household chores—by eating a little less. See Chapter 8 if you would like to try a model weight loss program.

Some Questions and Answers about Body Composition

▪ Can exercise reduce fat in particular parts of the body?

No. Most authorities reject the concept of "spot reduction." Stored fat belongs to the whole body, not just to the area where it happens to be stored. When you

YOUR FITNESS PROFILE 4-1
Estimated Calorie Costs of Your Fitness Activities

Objective: To calculate how many calories you use per week doing fitness activities.

Directions: The table lists calorie costs for a sampling of fitness activities included in Appendix B. The second column shows estimated costs of calories per minute per pound of body weight. Multiply your body weight by the figure in the second column to get your estimated calorie cost per minute for an exercise or activity. (Turn to Appendix B for other activities.) To determine the number of calories you expend each week in a fitness activity, multiply this figure by the number of minutes you engage in the activity in a week.

Calorie Cost for Selected Fitness Activities

Activity	Cal./min./lb.	× body weight	× min.	= Activity cal.
Aerobic dance (vigorous)	.062			
Basketball (vigorous, full court)	.097			
Bicycling (13 mph)	.071			
Canoeing (flat water, 4 mph)	.045			
Cross-country skiing (8 mph)	.104			
Handball (skilled, singles)	.078			
Horseback riding (trot)	.052			
Jogging (5 mph)	.060			
Rowing (vigorous)	.097			
Running (8 mph)	.104			
Soccer (vigorous)	.097			
Swimming (55 yds./min.)	.088			
Table tennis (skilled)	.045			
Tennis (beginner)	.032			
Walking (4.5 mph)	.048			
Other (from App. B or Model Programs)				
Other				
Other				
Total per week				

Rating: Estimated calories you expend in fitness activities per week: _____.

YOUR FITNESS PROFILE 4-2
Estimated Calorie Costs of Your Nonsport Activities

Objective: To calculate how many calories you use each week doing nonsport activities.

Directions: This table lists calorie costs for a sampling of nonsport activities. The second column shows estimated costs of calories per minute per pound of body weight. Multiply your body weight by the figure in the second column to get your estimated calorie cost per minute for an activity. To determine the number of calories you expend each week in a nonsport activity, multiply this figure by the number of minutes you engage in the activity in a week.

Calorie Cost for Selected Nonsport Activities

Activity	Cal./min./lb.	× body weight	× min.	= Activity cal.
Bathing, dressing, undressing	.021	_____	_____	_____
Bed-making (and stripping)	.031	_____	_____	_____
Chopping wood	.049	_____	_____	_____
Cleaning windows	.024	_____	_____	_____
Driving a car	.020	_____	_____	_____
Gardening				
Digging	.062	_____	_____	_____
Hedging	.034	_____	_____	_____
Raking	.024	_____	_____	_____
Weeding	.038	_____	_____	_____
Ironing	.029	_____	_____	_____
Kneading dough	.023	_____	_____	_____
Laundry (taking out and hanging)	.027	_____	_____	_____
Mopping floors	.024	_____	_____	_____
Painting house (outside)	.034	_____	_____	_____
Plastering walls	.023	_____	_____	_____
Sawing wood (crosscut saw)	.058	_____	_____	_____
Shoveling snow	.052	_____	_____	_____
Other (estimate from above)	____	_____	_____	_____
Other	____	_____	_____	_____
Other	____	_____	_____	_____
Total per week				

Rating: Estimated calories you expend in nonsport activities per week: _____.

YOUR FITNESS PROFILE 4-3
Estimated Calorie Costs of Your Sedentary Activities

Objective: To calculate how many calories you expend weekly in sedentary activities.

Directions: The table lists calorie costs for a sampling of sedentary activities. The second column shows estimated costs of calories per minute per pound of body weight. Multiply your body weight by the figure in the second column to get your estimated calorie cost per minute for an activity. To determine the number of calories you expend each week in a sedentary activity, multiply this figure by the number of minutes you engage in the activity in a week.

Calorie Cost for Selected Sedentary Activities

Activity	Cal./min./lb.	$\times$ body weight	$\times$ min.	= Activity cal.
Card playing	.012			
Eating (sitting)	.011			
Knitting and sewing	.011			
Piano playing	.018			
Sitting quietly	.009			
Sleeping and resting	.008			
Standing quietly	.012			
Typing (electric)	.013			
Writing	.013			
Other (estimate additional sedentary activities guided by the above list)				
Other				
Other				
Total per week				

Rating: Estimated calories you expend in sedentary activities per week: _____.

exercise, fat is mobilized from *all* the fat cells of the body. Spot exercising may build muscle in a specific area and thus may firm it up. But there is no evidence that the fat itself will disappear.

CRE exercise is best for losing weight. It uses more and larger muscle groups, and thus burns more calories, than brief localized exercise of individual parts of the body. Again, losing weight is a matter of patience and perseverance. A nutritionally sound diet together with a CRE program designed to achieve a negative calorie balance will help you lose weight, and you're sure—eventually—to lose some fat on your hips or around your waist.

Will a rubber exercise suit, vibrating machine, massage, or sauna help you lose weight?

A rubber exercise suit is useless for weight reduction, despite claims that it will help you sweat off fat. And after you've had a glass or two of fluid, even the loss of the fluid would not be sustained. In fact, dressing too warmly for exercise—which would include wearing a rubber suit—could even harm you as a result of dehydration.

Vibrators, massage, and saunas are just as ineffective for weight loss as rubber suits. An effective weight control program, as you know, requires activities that expend calories.

Advocates of the rubber suit and the sauna for weight loss also forget (or overlook) the fact that the body burns more calories when it's cool. If you exercise in a cool environment you would burn calories, which are units of heat, just to maintain your body temperature at 98.6°F. Therefore, the cooler the environment when you exercise, the more calories you're likely to expend.

Does weight training contribute to weight loss?

Because weight training is an excellent exercise for muscle development, it will increase the percentage of muscle in your body composition at the expense of the fat. To lose weight, use weight training to supplement an activity high in caloric expenditure, such as walking, jogging, running, swimming, or bicycling. These activities, which can be sustained over a long duration, burn many calories; if repeated regularly, they should help you lose weight. Combined with weight training, they give you a balanced program leading to a loss of fat and an increase in muscle.

Can exercise and diet help you gain weight?

By applying the same principle of calorie balance that works for weight reduction, you can also adjust your calorie intake to exceed your energy expenditure. Just as a negative calorie balance will cause you to lose weight, so a positive calorie balance will cause you to gain. Increase your dietary intake by 500 calories each day, and you should be able to gain one pound in two weeks. If your activity level goes up, you can eat more—and be sure that you eat enough so that you don't burn more calories than you take in.

Because most people prefer to put on lean, muscular weight rather than flab or fat, and because muscle is more dense than fat, you should try to increase your body's total muscle mass. Begin by following the basic weight training model program in Chapter 7, but use fewer repetitions for each exercise. By doing only 6 to 10 repetitions, you will stimulate muscle growth without burning too many calories. If you're also interested in increasing your CRE, be careful to do no more than the minimum requirements for a CRE program. And, once again, be sure that you do not burn more calories than you take in.

What happens to your muscles if you give up exercise?

Once you become inactive, the process of deconditioning begins: Muscle tissue is gradually lost. And fat is added if you continue to eat at the same levels as when you were physically active. Because one pound of fat is several times the volume of one pound of muscle, you'll probably notice a change in body composition even if you're able to maintain your weight.

Is it safe for an obese and sedentary person to begin an exercise program for weight reduction?

Yes, subject to the medical guidelines in Chapter 1. Getting started slowly is important for anyone who begins a new conditioning program. In this case, it would be crucial to use a program designed to begin with a very low overload. You may lose no weight at all for the first few weeks because muscles and the cardiorespiratory system will need some time to adjust to the new loads. You must be able to sustain a high enough level of activity for a long enough time before you can begin to burn those extra calories and shed fat. Patience is the most important element when you begin this kind of program. After the first few weeks, you should make significant and steady progress.

As we warned earlier in the chapter, resist the lure of crash diets. Weight loss on a crash diet is actually loss of fluid in most cases. It can be rapid but almost inevitably will not be maintained. A more gradual approach to weight loss—aiming for a maximum of one pound a week—will increase your chance of a permanent weight loss.

Can you do anything else besides diet and exercise to change body composition?

Yes, a formal exercise program is not the only way you can increase your expenditure of energy. You can burn extra calories by avoiding many conveniences that make life unnecessarily easy. Take the stairs instead of the elevator if you have only a few flights to climb. Park your car two or three blocks from your destination. Better still, leave your car at home and bike or walk as much as possible. Walk briskly instead of strolling. In short, survey your habits. Perhaps there are ways in which you can go a little farther and work a little harder if you forgo some step-saving and labor-saving "improvements." Altering your lifestyle in such seemingly insignificant ways can make a considerable difference—not only in weight control but in body composition and CRE as well—if you do it consistently over a long period of time.

Is it necessary to exercise within your EBZ as part of a weight control program?

Calories are expended at a lower rate per minute when you exercise below your EBZ. But since lower intensity activity can usually be continued for a longer period, you may actually burn more calories by the end of your workout. The more calories you burn, the more effective your weight control program will be.

If people weigh the same at age 65 as they did in college, doesn't that mean they have remained physically fit?

Not necessarily. Body weight is not a reliable measure of fitness. As explained in Chapter 1, body weight does not always accurately reflect whether you are fat. (Your weight could seem to be on the high side because you are heavily muscled, for example.) And even if you have maintained favorable body composition since your college days, you may still be less than fit in the other four fitness components. To find out how fit you are, assess your CRE, muscular strength, muscular endurance, and flexibility, as well as your body composition, following the suggestions in Chapter 1.

Does the ratio of fat to muscle necessarily increase as a person ages?

In general, the percentage of body fat does increase with advancing age. But it is impossible to know how much of this increase is due to the aging process and how much is due to atrophy of muscle tissue because of declining activity. It is true that people who continue to exercise into and beyond middle age do maintain leaner bodies than do sedentary people. But since even active people gain some fat as they grow older, it would be wise to cut back on calories. As activity levels decline, older people should adjust caloric intake to caloric output.

How are anorexia nervosa and bulimia related to an extreme fear of weight gain?

Some individuals, usually females, are extremely fearful of food and body fat; they relentlessly pursue being thin. This obsession with thinness, characterized by phobic behavior toward weight gain and food, is categorized as a disorder called *anorexia nervosa.*

Anorectic individuals may resort to extreme methods to stay slim or lose weight. Starvation, forced vomiting, or the constant use of laxatives are typical. Because of strong social pressures to eat, anorectics may indulge in deceptions to hide their extreme dieting from others. They may feed their food to the dog, flush it down the toilet, or throw it into the garbage. They offer any number of excuses for not eating. Even though anorectics may be lean or even emaciated, they remain terrified of becoming fat. In efforts to burn calories and lose weight, they may exercise enthusiastically to the point of marked hyperactivity.

One variation of anorexia is called *bulimia.* Bulimics gorge themselves for a period of time and later induce vomiting. The food binge–vomiting cycle may last for hours with a number of vomiting episodes. Initially, bulimics may feel relieved that they have found a way to eat and still maintain a low weight; however, they may become compulsive about the need to vomit and find that they can no longer control it voluntarily. In this extreme, hospitalization is necessary.

Anorexia and bulimia are complicated disorders usually connected to a variety of emotional and physical ills. They cannot be ignored and usually require the attention of experienced specialists.

5

Muscular Strength, Muscular Endurance, and Flexibility

After you've read this chapter, you will be able to:

Differentiate between muscular strength and endurance.

Recognize how muscles and nerves work together in strength and endurance activities.

Recognize how muscle use or disuse influences muscular atrophy and hypertrophy.

Differentiate among isotonic, isometric, and isokinetic muscular contractions and their various advantages.

Identify how you can use weight training to develop muscular strength and endurance.

Differentiate between weight training and weight lifting.

Recognize various myths connected with weight training.

Identify the role of calisthenics in developing muscular strength.

Recognize problems connected with strength and endurance development.

Recognize how flexibility serves to prevent muscular and joint problems.

Differentiate between the relative advantages of static versus ballistic stretching.

If you're like most people, you probably pay little attention to the condition of your muscles, tendons, ligaments, and joints. During a typical day, you make demands on your body that it can meet quite comfortably. Only when the demand is unusual, or when an injury occurs, are you likely to become aware of the strength, endurance, and flexibility of your musculoskeletal system. Your car's power steering conks out, and you struggle to turn the wheel. Or you write thirty thank-you notes after a birthday party and you're left with writer's cramp. Or after climbing fifteen flights of stairs during a power failure, your muscles become so sore that the next day you can hardly walk across the room. Worse still, an accident leaves you so weak that you can't sit up or even turn over in bed. All these examples of physical unfitness are caused, in large part, by personal limitations in the components known as muscular strength, muscular endurance, and flexibility.

MUSCULAR STRENGTH AND ENDURANCE

If you have difficulty turning the lid of an ordinary jar, opening a window that's stuck, or lifting a heavy suitcase onto a closet shelf, it's probably the result of inadequate muscular strength. In Chapter 1 we defined muscular strength as the ability to exert maximum force, usually in a single exertion (as when you lift a heavy weight). But muscular strength can have less clear-cut applications. Weak abdominal muscles, for example, may contribute to low-back pain, just as weak thigh muscles may increase the chances of injuring your knee. And you need muscular strength to support the weight of your body against the pull of gravity. Even when you sit in a chair, your muscles are exerting force on various parts of your skeleton without your consciously thinking about it. When muscular strength falls below minimal levels, you may even begin to experience difficulty getting up from a chair, climbing one or two steps, or performing the lightest of your routine tasks.

In general, your muscular strength is considered adequate if it lets you do your daily routine comfortably. Muscular strength is usually not an end in itself, but a way to achieve success and satisfaction from whatever physical activities you choose. (For those interested in competitive sports, of course, muscular strength is essential.) In short, muscular strength is basic to everything we do.

Muscular endurance is the ability to repeat a muscle contraction against resistance over and over again or to hold a particular muscle in a contracted position for an extended time. Posture, for example, may require more endurance than strength. Obviously, muscular endurance depends to some extent on muscular strength. Your muscles cannot repeat an action if they're too weak to perform it in the first place. Your muscular endurance also depends to some extent on your level of cardiorespiratory endurance (CRE). You cannot repeat an action many times over if your CRE cannot support the prolonged effort.

All body movements, including how you sit or stand, are brought about by the force of muscles pulling on tendons attached to bones. At every joint, opposing pairs of muscles coordinate to either flex or extend the joint. Some contract while others relax to bring about motion or to maintain position. In walking, for example, one

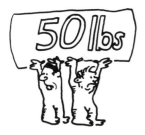 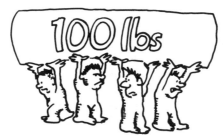

It takes more motor units of muscle fibers to lift heavier weights. As you develop more strength, you increase the size, not the number, of individual muscle fibers; the number of motor units you have remains constant through your life.

group of muscles on the front of the thigh (the hip flexors) pulls the thigh bone forward while a group on the back of the thigh (the hip extensors) relaxes to permit the thigh to move forward. For the next step, the flexors relax and the extensors contract so the one leg moves rearward as the other leg steps forward, and so on, as you walk. It's the central nervous system that coordinates the muscles by orchestrating the contractions and relaxations at the precise moment to ensure that movements are made smoothly.

Each muscle is composed of numerous individual *muscle fibers,* which are grouped in *motor units* consisting of all the muscle fibers supplied by a single nerve. The number of muscle fibers in a motor unit may vary from as few as five and up to fifty in muscles used for typing to as many as a thousand in muscles used for running. In each motor unit, the contraction of muscle fibers is triggered by an impulse from a nerve connected to the spinal cord and the higher centers of the central nervous system. When the muscle fibers in a motor unit contract, the force exerted by the motor unit is always the same: All the muscle fibers in the motor unit contract, and they contract maximally (they are incapable of partial contractions). The force exerted by the whole muscle, however, varies with the number of motor units called into action. If you lift fifty pounds, for instance, you use fewer motor units than if you lift one hundred pounds. Training improves the ability to call upon motor units to exert force. Training increases the rate that motor units are activated and coordinate their contraction. Most improvements in strength during the first two months of training and due to an improved ability to use motor units.

Although there is evidence in some animals that muscle fibers have adapted to severe work loads by increasing in number, this phenomenon, known as *hyperplasia,* has not yet been observed in humans. Until there is conclusive evidence to the contrary, we will continue to believe that the number of muscle fibers you have does not change over your lifetime. But the individual muscle fibers can change in size, depending on how you use your muscles. The more you use a particular muscle, the larger and stronger its individual muscle fibers become, especially with resistance exercise such as weight training. An increase in muscle size is called muscle *hypertrophy.* A decrease in muscle size, muscle *atrophy,* occurs if muscle fibers are not used enough or if the nerve supplying them is injured. The body does not maintain a muscle or nerve if you no longer use it or if it becomes immobilized.

A case in point is the experience of a young Air Force sergeant who had been run over by a truck. Seriously injured, he had to remain in a full body cast for about six months—a very long period to be inactive. By the time his cast was removed and he came under the care of a physical reconditioning facility, the sergeant had lost more than 120 pounds. Formerly a basketball player on an Air Force team, he found he couldn't even raise his arms. He looked more like a concentration camp inmate than a patient who had been medically cared for in a hospital. His was a classic case of muscle atrophy due to prolonged inactivity.

The early stages of the sergeant's reconditioning consisted of passive exercise: Therapists helped him raise his arms and legs. Within a few days he could raise his own arms and even feed himself. A week later, he was using light weights to exercise his upper extremities while lying in bed. Gradually, he became able to do partial sit-ups. After two weeks, he was wheeled each day to the gymnasium where he progressed to exercises in a wheelchair or on a bench. He continued to improve with a reconditioning program based on weight training. As he became able to lift heavier and heavier weights, his body weight began to increase. Fitted with a leg brace, he learned how to walk with crutches. By his third month of recovery, he had gained fifty pounds—and he reported that his upper body had become stronger than it had ever been.

To the sergeant, the improvement appeared almost miraculous, but to the rehabilitation staff it was not very remarkable. By repeatedly using his muscles, the sergeant was causing individual muscle fibers to become larger and stronger. By progressively making greater and greater demands on specific muscle groups, he was gradually increasing muscular strength. His muscles increased in size and weight, his body weight increased, and he improved in all aspects of fitness. The sergeant's successful rehabilitation program had made use of the two basic training principles: specificity—selection of appropriate activities to achieve selected fitness goals; and progressive overload—increasing the work by gradually adding to the intensity, duration, and frequency of the exercise program.

Isotonics, Isometrics, and Isokinetics

You can improve your muscular strength and endurance with an exercise program using any one of three types of muscular contractions. The first occurs in any activity in which there is movement. For example, lifting a weight, as the sergeant did, involves *isotonic* muscular contractions. To lift a weight, you contract your biceps muscle, causing your elbow to bend; your forearm moves, and you lift the weight in your hand.

The second type of contraction takes place when a muscle contracts without shortening and therefore without movement. Any exercise against an immovable resistance is known as *isometric* exercise. If you place your palms against a wall and push as hard as you can, keeping your elbows bent, your muscles contract but without causing movement in the joint or limb. With isometrics, gains in muscular strength are limited, occurring only at the point of contraction. Weight training, as a form of isotonic exercise, has been compared with isometrics. Although both methods contribute to strength development, weight training has the advantage of producing strength throughout the full range of movement. This also maintains flexibility. Isometric exercise, however, can develop muscular strength in a limb that is in a cast where range of movement is limited.

A third type of contraction is called *isokinetic*. Here movement takes place as in an isotonic contraction. But unlike isotonics, where the resistance remains fixed (as with the weight you lift), the speed of movement is constant and the resistance changes in response to the muscle group's maximal ability to exert force at various points throughout the range of motion.

Prospects are promising for isokinetic exercise. One of its advantages in fitness training is that the speed of movement during the exercise can be made to simulate speeds specific to various sports. What's more, the risk of muscle and joint injury is less and there is little or no muscle soreness resulting from isokinetic exercise. For most people, however, isokinetic exercise is not yet readily available.

Weight Training

If your primary fitness goal is to improve muscular strength and endurance, a weight training program should give you the benefits you seek, along with improvements in flexibility and body composition as well. Even CRE benefits can be worked on during weight training if you use light weights and many repeat lifts (repetitions) to increase duration. (See, for example, the interval circuit training model program in Chapter 7.)

Weight training is exercise using barbells and dumbbells (free weights) or machines offering comparable resistance, with weights and repetitions increased according to a specific overload system. The program is often referred to as progressive weight training (see Chapter 7 for a description of a model program). The equipment for weight training—barbells or dumbbells or both—is readily available and moderate in cost. For those who can afford it, more elaborate equipment is usually available at some fitness centers.

One caution before you begin a program of weight training. Because blood circulation tends to be impeded during weight training (and especially with isometrics), you should not undertake such a program without close medical supervision if you have a history of coronary heart disease, circulatory problems, or hypertension (high blood pressure). However, increased strength can benefit individuals with hypertension because the blood pressure response to a muscle load is less in people who are stronger.

By adjusting the amount of weight lifted and the number of repetitions, weight training can be adapted to emphasize either muscular strength or endurance. Heavy resistance with few repetitions works best for development of muscular strength. Light resistance with many repetitions is the key to muscular endurance.

An effective weight training program can be designed to supplement a general fitness program, one that includes aerobic training and flexibility workouts as well. Because it's important to start any new exercise program cautiously, begin weight training with light resistance for just a few repetitions until you've mastered the exercise. Increase your work load gradually over the weeks. Despite such precautions, your muscles may feel sore after a workout. You can obtain some relief by gently

TABLE 5-1   Weight Training Intensity

Goal	Range of repetitions
Muscular strength	6–8
Muscular endurance	15–25
Combination of muscular strength and muscular endurance	8–15

stretching the affected muscle. As with any exercise, of course, it's essential to warm up and cool down (see stretching model program in Chapter 7).

Studies show that when you use a weight that can be lifted at maximum effort, about 6 to 8 repetitions are effective for increasing muscular strength. With that regimen, once you're able to perform 8 repetitions, add to the resistance by switching to a heavier weight and return to 6 repetitions. To improve muscular endurance, about 15 to 25 repetitions appear to be beneficial. And once you handle 25 repetitions in a muscular endurance program, switch to a heavier weight to increase resistance and begin once again at 15 repetitions. To be equally balanced for muscular strength and muscular endurance, use a system of 8 to 15 repetitions with as much weight as you can handle. After you have achieved 15 repetitions, increase the weight and start with 8 repetitions. For best results, do 3 sets of repetitions every other day. See Table 5-1 for a summary of goals and repetitions.

A basic program in weight training can be adapted to meet special needs and individual goals. You may want to design a weight training program to improve your performance in a particular sport. For example, if golf is your game, you would want to build muscular strength in your wrists and forearms as well as in the trunk muscles. Because golf does not require much muscular endurance, you would need to do only 6 or 8 repetitions of the weight training exercise you select. Swimmers would work for muscular strength and for endurance of the muscles of the chest, shoulders, upper back, and thighs. For most swimmers, 8 to 15 repetitions of a weight training exercise would be appropriate.

What does weight training accomplish?

Most people use weight training to develop muscular strength and endurance as well as to improve muscle tone and physical appearance. Many also use weight training as a means of strengthening muscles and joints to minimize the chance of injury in competitive sports. Others use it to overcome an orthopedic problem, to prevent recurrence of one, or as part of an overall fitness and weight control program.

How does weight training differ from weight lifting?

A competitive sport, *weight lifting* is an event in which the person lifting the greatest amount of weight wins. Weight lifters compete against each other according to body weight classifications, as boxers do. Each weight lifter gets three attempts at each of the two lifts that make up the competition. In the two-hand snatch, the athlete brings the weight up from the floor in one quick movement to a straight-arm overhead position. In the clean-and-jerk, which permits the use of heavier weights, the weight is first brought to the chest and then lifted overhead. The score is the sum of the greatest weight lifted in each of the two lifts.

Weight training is not a competitive sport. True, some weight trainers are also interested in competitive *body building,* which emphasizes the development of large, well-defined muscles. Competitive body builders—sometimes called "iron pumpers"—however, strive for a degree of muscular hypertrophy far beyond what most noncompetitive weight trainers regard as desirable. Weight training should be viewed as a means toward achieving a goal, not an end in itself. Its goals are to increase muscular strength and endurance and to improve physique.

Can women undertake weight training?

Certainly. Women can respond as effectively to weight training as men to increase their general muscular strength and endurance and to prepare specific muscles for sports or other activities. In one supervised exercise program, untrained women, after a ten-week weight training program, were able to achieve greater increases in strength than the untrained men in the program.

Angie is a 19-year-old sophomore who works with weights to build herself up. She reports her muscles are firmer and better toned and claims that her increased strength has made her a better basketball and volleyball player. Melody, 29, wrote that she supplements "running by exercising with weights, which I have had at home for ten years. I can press sixty pounds easily, which is half my weight." She uses weights at least five days a week—"not long, just enough to increase my strength."

As these and many other women would attest, weight training does not lead to overmuscularization. The greater muscle mass in men is primarily the result of the male hormone testosterone. (This hormone is also present in women but not at the level found in men.) Furthermore, the increase in strength that both men and women obtain from weight training is not entirely due to increased muscle size. To some extent it comes from an increase in the number of motor units activated during a muscle's contraction. If you use a weight training program to bring more muscles into play, you can get a threefold increase in strength without getting a threefold increase in the size of your muscles. And once you develop your muscles to suit you, you can decrease the intensity of your workout (by decreasing the size of the weights, for example) to maintain rather than increase muscle size.

How does weight training affect body weight?

Because weight training develops your muscles, it will increase the percentage of your body composition that is muscle.

Does this mean that someone interested in *reducing* body weight should avoid weight training? Not necessarily. To lose body fat—but not muscle—choose activities likely to burn plenty of calories if you sustain them over a long duration. If you jog, walk, swim, or bicycle, for example, you could count on losing weight over a period of time. If you supplement these activities with weight training, you will lose fat while gaining muscle.

If you want to *gain* weight, you should supplement your training program with a high-calorie diet. As your muscle size increases, your body weight will increase.

■   **At what age can a youngster begin weight training?**

It's safe to begin weight training in early adolescence, as soon as a boy or girl shows interest in the activity. The idea that weight training can cause hernia, muscle-boundness, and heart damage has long been refuted. Quite the contrary. Controlled studies, including one with forty-six boys from 12 to 17 years of age, have not shown any physical problems resulting from a program of weight training for young people.

Some youngsters may want to begin weight training when they see parents, older siblings, or friends enjoying benefits of muscle improvement—or just enjoying the activity of weight training itself. Others, like some of their elders, may be interested primarily in improving their musculature.

Many young people come to weight training to improve and maintain their strength and endurance in order to enhance their performance in competitive sports. Football players, gymnasts, runners, swimmers, and wrestlers often use weight training both in and out of season. An important advantage of weight training for younger as well as older athletes, in addition to improving sports performance, is the reduction of athletic injuries associated with improved muscular strength and endurance.

■   **How old is too old for weight training?**

You're never too old for weight training. Healthy people in their fifties, sixties, seventies, or older can benefit from a sound weight training program, but it should be used to supplement a regimen emphasizing CRE activities such as walking, jogging, swimming, or bicycling.

Muscles often lose their strength with aging, but a person can minimize or reverse these losses by regular weight training. The exercise, like any other, should be begun cautiously and increased slowly, especially by those who've been inactive. Beginning with light weights and few repetitions, older people can adjust gradually to the new activity. Weight training can be continued for as long as an older person is in reasonably good shape and has no cardiovascular problems.

■   **Does exercise increase a woman's bust?**

Exercise cannot increase bust size, but it can strengthen the muscles supporting the breasts—and that can change appearance. To strengthen these muscles, a woman should select three or four exercises for the pectoral muscles, located on the front of her chest, and do the exercises for 8 to 15 repetitions every other day.

Calisthenics

Compared with weight training, calisthenics is less likely to help as much with muscular strength as with muscular endurance. But you can use push-ups, sit-ups, and other calisthenics if weight training is not available or desirable.

If you can't do even a single push-up on the floor, begin a program in calisthenics by doing a push-up against the wall. (See Figure 5-1.) Work up to 15 repetitions. Then work up to 15 repetitions using a table for support, and then switch to a chair. After that, you should be ready for the floor. At each stage you would use the three-set system—doing each set of repetitions three times every other day.

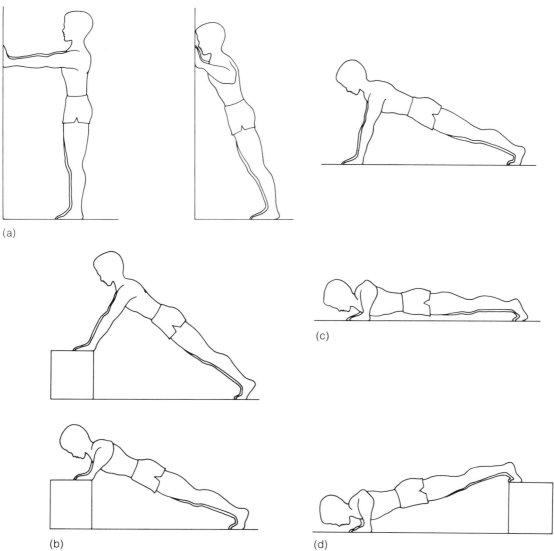

FIGURE 5-1   Push-up variations. The easiest way to do them is against a wall (a). Stand a straight-arm's distance away from the wall. Keeping your back and legs straight and your feet on the floor, lean forward until your nose touches the wall. Then push your body back into a vertical position. Next advance to the elevated push-up (b). First use a table (in place of the wall), then a chair, then an object lower than a chair—say, a box or footstool. Finally, try the traditional floor position (c). To add resistance, raise your feet and then lower your chest to the floor (d).

You can use an adjustable slant board as an aid in learning how to do sit-ups. (See Figure 5-2.) Many sedentary people have mastered the sit-up by following this procedure. To begin, set the angle of elevation of the slant board fairly high. Position yourself on the slant board with your feet at the lower end. Try for a minimum of 6 repetitions and continue at that angle until you can do 15. Then lower the angle a bit

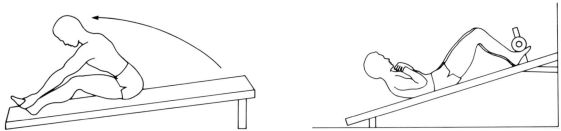

FIGURE 5-2   Sit-ups using a slant board. If you can't do even one sit-up, start with your head at the high end of the board. As the sit-ups become easier, gradually lower the head of the board until you are doing sit-ups on a level surface. You can increase resistance by doing sit-ups with your head at the lower end of the slant board. Always perform these exercises with your knees bent.

and follow the same pattern of repetitions. Do this each time you lower the angle of the slant board until you can perform 15 sit-ups on a flat board. (Once again, use the three-set system for best results.) Once you have achieved this, you will want to place your head at the low end for adequate resistance.

Some Cautions

Calisthenics, like weight training, is safe for those who qualify under our medical guidelines in Chapter 1. But, as we've said, people with coronary heart disease or coronary risk factors, circulatory problems, or hypertension should consult a physician before beginning such programs. The increase in blood pressure that occurs during the exercise program may be risky, and you should observe other cautions as well.

Muscular Training and Orthopedic Problems   Whether you rely on weight training or calisthenics to build up muscular strength and endurance, proceed cautiously if you have any orthopedic difficulties. Having orthopedic problems, however, does not mean that you must, as a matter of course, avoid exercise. If the problems are localized—and they usually are—you can develop an exercise program around them. If the difficulties involve specific groups of muscles, bones, or joints, it is usually possible to design a program that avoids using the affected part or parts while strengthening the rest of the body.

If, for example, you are recuperating from knee surgery, you can perform upper-body exercises while you sit or lie down. You can also exercise the other leg. Indeed, exercise programs are often designed specifically to rehabilitate orthopedic disabilities. Obviously, such a program must be designed with your individual problems in mind. For example, exercises that place too much strain on the lower back would simply aggravate a lower-back condition.

Consider Barry, who suffered month-long backaches on and off for several years. Finally his physician advised him to undertake weight training to strengthen his lower back. He went to the college gym for his specific therapeutic workout.

While there, Barry decided he might as well try a complete three-day-a-week program. He wrote that after three years, "I have progressed to a six-day-a-week split routine (three days on legs, chest, and back alternated with three days on arms, shoulders, and abdominals)." As for the original orthopedic difficulty, Barry reported, "My back problems have gone away totally. . . . My original goal has been attained—no back pain."

No matter what your orthopedic condition, you should beware of lifting anything—whether a barbell or a suitcase—with your knees straight. Lifting from the floor should always be done with a straight back and bent knees, even by someone with no tendency to back weakness.

Exercises No One Should Do   Not all exercises are safe and sensible. You should avoid some no matter how much they may be touted as beneficial to you. Each of the following may lead to injury.

The full squat, when performed repetitively, can injure knee ligaments. It includes among its variations repeated deep-knee bends, duck waddling, and the Russian bounce. These exercises have you squat low with the buttocks touching the back of the lower leg or the heels (Figure 5-3).

The straight leg sit-up, performed with legs extended and held straight, tends to pull the vertebrae forward (Figure 5-4). It increases the possibility of lordosis ("swayback"), a contributing factor to low-back problems. Be wary of this exercise, which is sometimes claimed to strengthen the abdominal muscles. (The leg lift, also known as the leg raise, can cause some of the same problems as the straight leg sit-up.) Instead, do the bent knee sit-up, which places the workload more directly on the

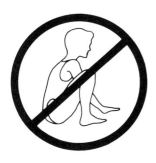

FIGURE 5-3   The full squat—an exercise to avoid. Alternative safe exercise: squat to position where thighs are parallel to floor.

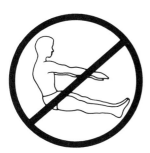

FIGURE 5-4   The straight-leg sit-up—an exercise to avoid. Alternative safe exercise: Bent-knee sit-up.

abdominal muscles. It is even more likely to do so if, when sitting up, you round your back until you reach the sit-up position.

In the straight-knee toe touch, you are supposed to bend over from a standing position, keeping your knees straight, and while bouncing try to touch the floor with your fingers (Figure 5-5). The back muscles would tend to be elongated, which would increase the possibility of "swayback" (see above).

The plow can injure the vertebrae of the neck as well as the lower back. Its benefits are outweighed by these potential hazards (Figure 5-6).

The hurdler's stretch, which is frequently used to stretch the hamstrings and the muscles of the groin, has been known to injure the knee ligaments of the rear leg (Figure 5-7). There are many safer exercises to choose from.

The bent-over rowing motion falls into a different category. This exercise can be safe—and beneficial—if performed with the proper precautions. If done incorrectly, however, it can lead to injury. We recommend that you do the bent-over row-

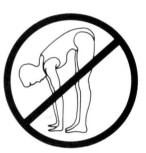

FIGURE 5-5   The straight-knee toe touch—an exercise to avoid. Alternative safe exercise: Do exercise in seated position with knees bent.

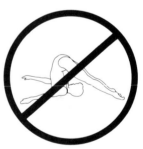

FIGURE 5-6   The plow—an exercise to avoid.

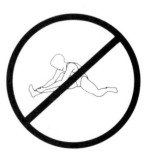

FIGURE 5-7   The hurdler's stretch—an exercise to avoid. Alternative safe exercise: See exercise 6, p. 141, in Chapter 7.

ing motion (which you do while standing) only with your forehead resting on a table or some other support and your knees bent to ease the strain on the lower back.

"Negative" Work and Muscle Soreness   Some exercise physiologists who have studied the "negative" phase of exercise—lowering yourself to the floor after pushing up, or lowering yourself after chinning up to a bar, or lowering to your chest a weight that you've lifted overhead—believe that it may contribute to muscle soreness. So-called negative work appears to be no less beneficial than the positive phase of exercise in contributing to training effects, although it is less fatiguing than positive exercise. But because of the possible association with muscle soreness, negative work should probably not be the primary focus of an exercise program.

A Warning to Weight Lifters   Anyone who lifts weights should observe one caution in particular. No matter how healthy you are, don't hold your breath during weight lifting. The rule is to inhale in preparation for the lift and exhale at the conclusion of the lift.

Even competitive weight lifters occasionally become light-headed from lifting an extremely heavy weight. The cause is a series of events, initiated during the lifting of weight, when a person tries to exhale with the epiglottis closed. (The epiglottis is a small flap of tissue deep in the throat; it prevents food or liquid from entering the windpipe.) The resulting increase in chest pressure activates the vagus nerve, which causes the heart to slow. That in turn may cause a drop in the blood flow to the brain to the point of light-headedness or even fainting.

FLEXIBILITY

The third musculoskeletal component of fitness is flexibility—the ability to flex and extend each joint through its normal range of motion. Flexibility in any joint depends on the condition of bones, tendons, ligaments, and muscles and on the interrelations of all these body parts. Joints that are regularly moved through their full range of motion and muscles that regularly flex and extend fully will retain full normal mobility.

Flexibility is not a single characteristic uniformly present in all parts of the body. Some of your joints are probably a lot more flexible than others. Bursitis may limit the flexibility of your shoulder. Or bicycling may have improved the flexibility of your knees. To test your normal range of motion, you will need to move various joints in specified ways. The examples in Profile 5-1 illustrate movements you can use to determine your flexibility for some of the important joints.

In the past it was believed that weight training could limit a person's flexibility and that strong people were likely to be muscle-bound. That myth has been laid to rest. Authorities now agree that flexibility is not impeded by weight training. In fact, champion weight lifters and body builders tend to be more flexible than average. It is true that activities that use only a limited range of motion in a particular muscle group may shorten the muscles involved. Jogging, for example, accentuates partial movements of muscle groups and so encourages tightening of the hamstring muscles, the

YOUR FITNESS PROFILE 5-1
Determining Your Normal Range of Joint Motion

Objective: To estimate the flexibility and range of motion in your major joints.

Directions: Illustrated here is the normal range of motion for some of the major joints. By comparing the motion of your joints with the illustrations, you should be able to determine whether you have normal range. The approximate degree of movement is noted on each illustration. If any one of your joints has a limited range, see the stretching model program in Chapter 7. If you decide to try to increase your range of motion, remember that for most people there is no need to achieve flexibility beyond normal range.

1. Raise and lower your arm at the shoulder, sideward.

    ____ Range OK

    ____ Needs
    Improvement

    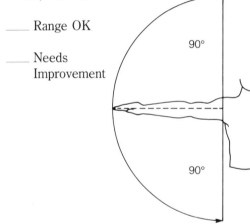

2. Turn your shoulder, palm outward and palm inward.

    ____ Range OK

    ____ Needs
    Improvement

    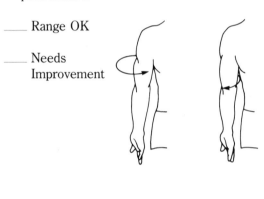

3. Raise and lower your arm at the shoulder, forward and to the rear.

    ____ Range OK

    ____ Needs
    Improvement

    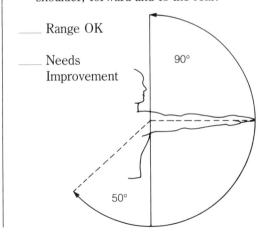

4. Turn your palm up and palm down.

    ____ Range OK

    ____ Needs
    Improvement

    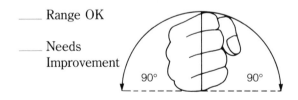

5. Bend and straighten your elbow.

___ Range OK

___ Needs
     Improvement

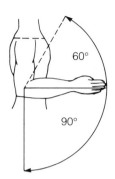

6. Raise leg to the side at the hip.

___ Range OK

___ Needs
     Improvement

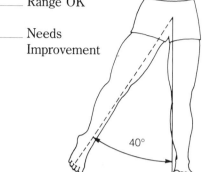

7. Raise and lower your leg forward at
   the hip.

___ Range OK

___ Needs
     Improvement

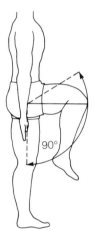

8. Bend and straighten your knee.

___ Range OK

___ Needs
     Improvement

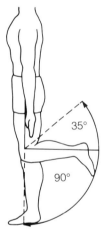

9. Raise and lower your foot at the ankle.

___ Range OK

___ Needs
     Improvement

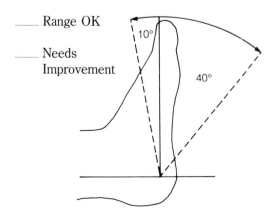

hip flexors (the muscles that bring the leg forward), and the quadriceps. But you can take steps to avoid the problem by supplementing your jogging with exercises designed to stretch those muscles. If you train with weights, you must be careful to keep your muscles flexible by performing each exercise correctly, moving through the full range of motion required. If you dance or do karate—exercises that promote flexibility—you probably already enjoy high levels of flexibility.

It is possible that improving flexibility may improve strength in certain muscle groups. This is due to the principle of reciprocal inhibition: As a muscle contracts to near its normal range of motion, it is turned off by stretch receptors in the opposing muscle group. In the leg, for example, the quadriceps (the muscles on the front of the thigh) are inhibited from contracting further as stretch receptors in the hamstrings (the muscles on the back of the thigh) are stimulated. In someone with tight hamstrings, the quadriceps are turned off prematurely, which lessens their ability to improve their strength. Improving flexibility may make it possible to more easily increase strength during weight training and other forms of exercise.

Regaining lost flexibility is a slow process but well worth the time and effort. Persistence may pay off in marked improvement in flexibility. In working for flexibility, it's pointless to try to exceed the normal range of motion. In fact, extreme flexibility—loose-jointedness—is of no particular benefit and may even lead to stretched ligaments and weakness in some joints.

Anyone exercising to improve CRE or muscular fitness can benefit from flexibility training too. It is particularly well suited to the warm-up and cool-down periods. It can also help ease the pain and discomfort that may result from efforts to return to normal activity after an illness or a sedentary vacation. Flexibility training can also help overcome soreness after overdoing activities—overexertion on your first ski outing of the season, say. It can also help counter the ill effects of sitting at a desk all day (shortening the hamstrings), wearing high-heeled shoes (shortening the Achilles tendon), or simply getting older.

Jason wrote, "I have to do regular stretching exercises to leave me flexible and decrease problems with tendonitis and lower-back aches and pains. After I learned about the need for flexibility exercise, I have performed it regularly (every day) and tried to do it right before handball, tennis, jogging, cycling, or skiing. . . . The sessions only require about fifteen minutes or less."

The best way to develop flexibility is to use stretching exercises, and the best way to stretch is slowly and gradually, using a technique called *static stretching*. See stretching model program in Chapter 7.

■ Why is gradual stretching preferred over bouncing?

Gradual or "static" stretching is a technique in which you achieve positions slowly and hold them passively for a few seconds up to as much as a minute. Bouncing or bobbing, called "ballistic" stretching, is characterized by the momentum of bouncing movements that are designed to force the muscles into a greater stretch.

Although research has shown little difference in the effectiveness of these two methods, static stretching offers less risk of injury due to overstretching, and it doesn't seem to result in sore muscles. In fact, people often use static stretching to relieve muscle soreness caused by exercise. Bouncing may cause the muscles being stretched to contract defensively, thereby resulting in the shortening of the muscles.

What is the relationship between flexibility and sports performance?

The ability to stretch throughout the normal range of motion is a useful ability for athletes and dancers. The greater freedom of movement flexibility provides enhances the ability to reach and stretch during performance. Activities that require easy movement from one position to another while bending, leaping, and reaching include tennis, racquetball, handball, downhill skiing, gymnastics, and most team sports.

Good flexibility is also essential in preventing sports injuries. Extreme looseness in the joints, erroneously referred to as "double-jointedness," is not desirable, however, and may contribute to an excessive risk of dislocation from stretched ligaments.

Why do you recommend warming up before stretching?

It is a good idea to precede stretching with a brief warm-up such as jogging in place for several minutes. The rise in muscle temperature resulting from the increased blood flow helps improve muscle elasticity. Stretching after an aerobic or strength workout is also helpful both for maintaining and improving flexibility and reducing the risk of muscle soreness.

How does inactivity contribute to poor flexibility?

When a joint is not regularly moved through its complete range of motion, a shortening of the muscles usually results. An extreme example of this phenomenon is seen when a cast is removed from an arm or leg after five or six weeks. Not only will the muscles appear weak and atrophied, but the affected joint will be stiff and hard to move. Weeks of stretching and strengthening may be needed to regain the normal range of motion. In a less dramatic way, constant sitting in a chair with the hips and knees flexed as is natural will cause a tightness in the muscles that surround these joints.

6

Eating Right

After you've read this chapter, you will be able to:

Identify the essential nutrients and their primary sources and functions.

Decide whether you need to change your eating patterns to better adhere to recommended U.S. dietary goals and guidelines.

Plan nutritionally balanced menus that include foods from the daily food guide.

Recognize why it is prudent to limit your intake of salt, sugar, caffeine, saturated fats, and high-cholesterol foods in your diet.

Assess your need for food supplements.

Recognize common misconceptions related to eating and exercise.

The increased interest in fitness and weight control has been accompanied by concern about the need for adequate nutrition. Eating is clearly one of America's favorite activities; we spend billions each year to gorge ourselves at burgeoning fast-food chains. When we aren't busy shoveling in the food, we're thinking about our next meal. And how can we help it? The advertising media constantly remind us of the marvelous juicy burger on a huge, tasty bun and other delicious concoctions. Supermarket tabloids display vivid color photos and recipes of all kinds to tantalize our palates. At the same time, newsstands and magazine racks feature books and articles warning us about the hazards of overeating.

Some people, like Sandy, are understandably confused. "We are urged to use vitamin and mineral supplements, while at the same time we are being told that they are a waste of money." She went on to say, "I want to do what's best for me, but I don't know what that is." Kim's problem is different: "What with rushing to and from class and spending hours at a time in the lab, I don't have time to eat all that much." Instead, she grabs a quick burger and fries on the run. Despite this, she seems to be getting heavier.

In Chapter 4 we dealt with the principles of controlling fat. Here we present some nutrition basics to guide you in your food decision making.

NUTRIENTS

Proteins, carbohydrates, fats, vitamins, minerals, and water are the six categories of nutrients derived from food that fulfill three primary functions in the body:

- Providing energy
- Building and repairing body tissues
- Regulating body processes

Let's look at each of these nutrients and its specific roles.

Proteins

Proteins, the building blocks of the body, are ever changing and in perpetual need of replacement. Of the approximately twenty-two amino acids that make up protein, scientists consider nine essential because they cannot be synthesized in the body and must be provided by the foods we eat. Protein is found in both animal and plant sources. Only animal protein contains all the essential amino acids and is thus "complete." This could pose a problem for "vegans" who avoid eggs and milk products. But a person can overcome this problem by carefully combining plant sources at a given meal to supply complete proteins. Examples of how various ethnic groups have dealt with a lack of animal foods are: rice with beans, minestrone soup, and baked beans with brown bread.

While many people around the world, including some in the United States, suffer from a lack of protein, most Americans get enough protein in their regular diets;

and even with an increase in the amount of exercise, protein supplements aren't necessary. Any increase in your calorie intake will almost automatically raise the amount of protein in your diet.

Carbohydrates

Carbohydrates are among the cheapest sources of calories and therefore supply most of the world's human energy. Here in the energy-rich United States, carbohydrates are mistakenly believed to be both fattening and nutritionally poor. This unearned reputation could result from the idea that carbohydrates are primarily high-calorie candies, sweet desserts, soda, cereals, and other processed foods to which large amounts of refined sugar are added. Such high-calorie products deserve their reputation as "empty calorie" foods because they have little nutritional value other than the calories they contain. In contrast, naturally occurring sugars and starches found in plant foods are rich in nutrients.

Carbohydrates, with the exception of milk sugar, are virtually nonexistent in animal foods. The three major types of carbohydrate found in plants are

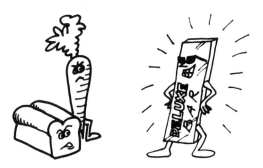

"He may look good, but he's really a good-for-nothing!"

- Sugars—simple carbohydrates
- Starches—complex carbohydrates
- Fiber—digestion-resistant carbohydrates (roughage)

Most nutritionists believe that we should be eating a greater proportion of unrefined complex carbohydrates. Not only are they essential as fuel for intensive activity, but they are also instrumental in sparing body protein as an energy source and allowing fats to be used more efficiently. Adequate glucose, from carbohydrate, must be readily available so that the brain and nervous system work properly.

Actually, we consume fewer carbohydrates today than we did earlier in the century—despite a large increase in the consumption of "empty-calorie" sweets. The decrease is apparently in the complex carbohydrates found naturally in grains, fruits, and vegetables.

Fats

Fats serve several important functions. Fats are packed with twice as much energy per unit of weight as either protein or carbohydrate and are valuable as an energy source during moderate physical activity. Because fat is slow to leave the stomach, eating foods high in fat (as many fast foods are) delays the feeling of hunger for pro-longed periods. (This is the reason that fast foods leave you feeling full for a long time after you have consumed them.) Fat also cushions the internal organs, insulates the body against cold, provides linoleic acid (a fatty acid not produced by the body), and carries fat-soluble vitamins. When caloric intake exceeds energy needs, protein and carbohydrate are converted into fat, which is stored in the body's fat cells. Once stored, this fat can later be mobilized into the bloodstream to serve as an energy source.

There are two types of fats or lipids: saturated fat, which comes primarily from animal sources as well as from palm, palm kernel, and coconut oils (used in processed foods), and unsaturated fat supplied by fruits, vegetables, and grains. Saturated fat is generally a solid, and unsaturated fat is a liquid or oil. It is important to note the difference. Saturated fats, which should be limited in the diet, are used by the body to manufacture cholesterol. Some foods that contain saturated fat may also contain cholesterol, infamous in its relationship with coronary artery disease. Unsaturated fats are cholesterol free, and, in fact, some monounsaturated and polyunsaturated fats can actually reduce the level of cholesterol in the blood.

Today we consume more fat—about 45 percent of our diet is fat—than we did in the year 1900. Most authorities believe that this percentage should be between 25 and 30 percent. Some insist it should be even lower.

Vitamins

Unlike proteins, carbohydrates, and fats, vitamins are not a source of energy. They are essential, however, for maintaining good health. If a vitamin is lacking, a specific problem or deficiency can occur. A familiar example is the lack of vitamin C that led to scurvy among British sailors in the days of sailing ships; adding citrus to the ships' fare overcame the problem. Vitamins fall into two groups: Vitamins A, D, E, and K are fat soluble, and vitamin C and the B-complex vitamins are water soluble (Table 6-1).

The question of whether vitamin supplements are routinely needed is a common one. The answer seems to be no unless your eating habits are poor or you have a specific problem. Anyone who eats a variety of foods is likely to be getting all the vitamins necessary. In spite of this, approximately 50 percent of all Americans spend millions of dollars per year on vitamin pills. Water-soluble vitamins are not stored in the body, and the excess is flushed out to become very expensive urine. "One multivitamin per day" makes some people feel good, however, and the practice doesn't seem to be dangerous.

Minerals

A nutritional mineral is a solid natural element essential to the sustenance of life. Two groups of minerals are required in the diet. Those with a daily requirement of more than 100 mg. are considered the major minerals, and those with a requirement of less than 100 mg. are known as trace minerals. Calcium and phosphorus located in the teeth and bones account for up to 85 percent of the body's mineral content.

TABLE 6-1   Vitamins

Vitamin	Source	Function
Fat soluble		
A	Liver, butter, cheese, margarine, milk, eggs, yellow vegetables and fruits, green leafy vegetables	Develops and maintains skin and mucous membranes, adaptation to dim light, tooth and bone development
D	Fortified dairy products, liver, sunlight, oily fish	Regulates calcium and phosphorus absorption, bone and tooth development
E	Cereals, wheat germ, nuts, legumes, vegetable oils, green leafy vegetables	Prevents oxidation of other vitamins and fatty acids
K	Liver, spinach, cauliflower, cabbage, egg yolks, soybean oil	Blood clotting
Water soluble		
B_1 (thiamine)	Milk, whole grain foods, meat, pork, liver, legumes, wheat germ, potatoes, nuts	Energy metabolism, growth
B_2 (riboflavin)	Milk, cheese, whole-grain foods, meat, eggs, fish, green leafy vegetables	Functioning of body tissues
Niacin	Lean meats, poultry, fish, liver, whole-grain foods, peanuts, legumes	Energy metabolism
B_6 (pyridoxine)	Whole-grain foods, meat, fish, poultry, legumes, milk	Protein metabolism, polyunsaturated fat metabolism
Pantothenic acid	Whole-grain foods, milk, cheese, legumes, broccoli, tomatoes, salmon, meat	Carbohydrate, fat, protein metabolism
Folicin	Meat, liver, milk, eggs, green leafy vegetables, oranges, legumes, broccoli, asparagus	Growth, normal cell division
Biotin	Meat, liver, eggs, legumes, fruits, vegetables, nuts	Carbohydrate, fat, protein metabolism
B_{12} (cobalamin)	Meat, poultry, fish, eggs, milk products	Functioning of all body cells
C	Citrus fruits, strawberries, tomatoes, melons, cabbage, potatoes, broccoli, peppers	Tissue repair, tooth and bone formation

Each mineral serves a specific function, and some serve several functions. A well-balanced diet of sufficient caloric content should supply enough of the essential minerals. (See Table 6-2.)

Water

Water, seldom thought of as a nutrient, composes about 60 percent of our body weight. Actually, water is the most important nutrient because it serves as the medium in which the other five nutrients function. In fact, water is a part of the body. It cools, acts as a cushion for nerves, lubricates the joints, removes waste products, and helps in digestion.

Although you can survive the loss of most body fat, carbohydrate, and protein, loss of about a tenth of your body's weight in water would probably end your life. Even temporary dehydration can result in severe physiological problems.

The body's daily need for water is normally slightly more than two quarts. With

TABLE 6-2   Minerals Found in Humans

Mineral	Source	Function
Major minerals		
Calcium	Milk products, leafy green vegetables, broccoli, shellfish	Bone and tooth formation, blood clotting, nerve transmission
Phosphorus	Milk, cheese, meat, fish, poultry, eggs, whole-grain foods, legumes, nuts	Acid-base balance, hormone regulation, energy production, bone formation
Magnesium	Whole-grain foods, legumes, nuts, green vegetables, meat, milk	Activates enzymes
Sodium	Salt, milk, seafood, eggs, bread	Regulation of body fluids, transfer of nutrients across cell walls
Potassium	Fruits, vegetables, meat, fish, poultry, cereals, legumes	Regulation of body fluids, transfer of nutrients across cell walls
Chlorine	Salt, seafood, eggs, milk, meat	Activates enzymes
Sulfur	Meat, milk, nuts, legumes	Formation of body tissues
Trace minerals		
Iron	Liver, meats, eggs, legumes, whole-grain foods, dried fruits, green leafy vegetables	Oxygen transport
Iodine	Iodized salt, seafood, vegetables	Helps form thyroxin
Copper	Meat, shellfish, liver, vegetables, cherries, legumes, poultry	Formation of enzymes
Zinc	Meat, poultry, fish, milk, vegetables, wheat bran	Component of various enzymes
Fluorine	Drinking water, seafood, green leafy vegetables	Reduces dental caries; formation of bones and teeth
Manganese	Whole-grain foods, leafy vegetables, legumes, fruit	Enzyme functions
Molybdenum	Whole-grain foods, legumes, green leafy vegetables, liver	In several enzymes
Selenium	Grains, onions, meat, fish, milk, vegetables	Fat metabolism
Chromium	Meat, vegetable oils, clams, whole-grain foods, water	Glucose metabolism

vigorous physical activity or high temperatures, you require more. It is prudent to drink plenty of fluids routinely—don't wait until you are thirsty.

NUTRITIONAL GUIDELINES

Alarmed by the population's trend toward greater consumption of fats and refined sugars and their detrimental effect on the nation's health, the U.S. Senate established a Select Committee on Nutrition and Human Need. This committee formulated "Dietary Goals for the United States," which are illustrated in Table 6-3. In general the Select Committee called for a reduction in the consumption of fats, refined sugar, cholesterol, and salt and an increase in the consumption of naturally occurring carbohydrates.

TABLE 6-3   Present Diet Versus U.S. Dietary Goals

	Current diet	Dietary goals
Fat	42%	30%
Saturated	16%	10%
Monounsaturated	13%	10%
Polyunsaturated	13%	10%
Carbohydrates	46%	58%
Simple	24%	10%
Complex	22%	48%
Protein	12%	12%

Note: Specifically, the "Dietary Goals" call for a 12 percent reduction in dietary fat, with saturated fat being limited to 10 percent of the total fat ingested. They recommend a 12 percent increase in total carbohydrates, but with an increase of 26 percent in complex carbohydrates (naturally occurring starches) and a 14 percent reduction in simple carbohydrates (sugars). Protein intake remains the same.

In an attempt to clarify these goals, the U.S. Department of Agriculture announced the following "dietary guidelines":

1. Eat a variety of foods.
2. Avoid excessive fat, saturated fat, and cholesterol.
3. Maintain ideal weight.
4. Eat foods adequate in starch and fiber.
5. Avoid too much sugar.
6. Avoid too much salt and sodium.
7. If you drink alcohol, do so in moderation.

The National Cholesterol Education Program, with the endorsement of thirty-eight federal agencies and health organizations, proposed new guidelines recommending an even lower intake of saturated fats than those suggested in the "Dietary Goals for the United States." These low-fat recommendations are depicted in Table 6-4. Although the new standard for total fat is similar to the previous recommendation, the new proposal for intake of saturated fat is "none."

A BALANCED DIET

The daily food guide evolved from an effort to classify into simple categories foods that resemble each other in nutritional content. When using it to plan your diet, it is important for you to keep the seven nutritional guidelines in mind when you select specific foods. For example, to lower your consumption of saturated fats and cholesterol, skimmed milk is a better choice than whole milk, and fish and poultry are

TABLE 6-4   New Low-fat Recommendations

	Recommended diet	Current diet*
Total fat	Average of 30% or less of daily calorie intake	36%–37%
Saturated	None	15%–16%
Polyunsaturated	Up to 10%	7%
Monounsaturated	Rest of fat calories	14%
Cholesterol	Less than 300 mg. a day	Women: 304 Men: 435

*Figures are for adults

SOURCE: *National Cholesterol Education Program* as reported in the *New York Times* (Feb. 28, 1990, p. A22).

TABLE 6-5   The Daily Food Guide

Group	Servings	Cautions
Fruit-vegetable	Four or more daily	Choose widely from among the varieties. Fresh is generally better
Bread-cereal	Four or more daily	Use mainly whole-grain or enriched products. Check on the contents of processed foods
Milk and milk products	Two or more daily	Use skim or low-fat versions
Meat, fish, eggs, poultry, beans	Two or more daily	Limit high-cholesterol foods such as eggs and red meat
Fats, sweets, and alcohol	See caution	Should not replace choices from the four groups above. Amounts consumed should be based on caloric need

wiser choices than red meat. To be certain your vitamin and mineral intakes are adequate, select widely from the bread and cereal group and the fruit and vegetable group. You will also have to do some interpreting. Pizza, for example, doesn't fit into a single group; the cheese, dough, and tomato sauce represent three separate food groups. And finally, your total calories should not exceed your daily energy demands. If they do, you will gradually gain weight.

In Chapter 4 we discussed the combined roles of diet and exercise in controlling body fat. When planning to reduce your caloric intake, it is important to adhere to the number of servings recommended in Table 6-5; to reduce your weight, reduce the size of your servings. This ensures a balanced diet. We present a step-by-step approach to weight control based on a balanced diet in Chapter 8, "Model Weight Loss Program." The information in Appendix C, "Food Exchange Plan," provides information to implement the program.

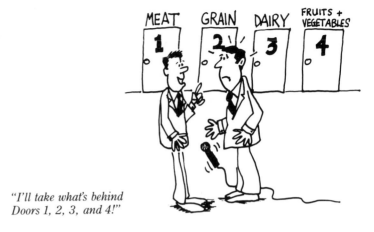

"I'll take what's behind Doors 1, 2, 3, and 4!"

QUESTIONS AND ANSWERS

What is wrong with tropical oils?

Although vegetable oils are predominantly unsaturated, tropical oils are an exception. Palm, palm kernel, and coconut oils are highly saturated and should be avoided. It is wise to avoid processed foods that contain these tropical oils because they are saturated fat from which the body manufactures cholesterol (Table 6-6).

Many of the standard baking and food processing companies have already responded to the demands for healthier ingredients by eliminating cholesterol from their products and by switching from tropical oils to other vegetable oils. It is wise to carefully read food labels so that you know what you are purchasing.

TABLE 6-6   Cholesterol Content of Selected Foods*

Meat, fish, and eggs	Mg.	Milk and milk products	Mg.
Liver (cooked, 3½ oz.)	438	Milk, whole (8 oz.)	34
Eggs (1 large)	252	Milk, skim (8 oz.)	5
Shrimp (10 small)	150	Cheese, American (1 oz.)	28
Lobster (3½ oz.)	85	Ice cream (1 cup)	85
Clams (10)	60	Ice milk (1 cup)	10
Veal (3½ oz.)	99	Butter (1 pat)	12
Pork (3½ oz.)	88	Cream cheese (1 tbsp.)	18
Beef (3½ oz.)	91	Cottage cheese (4 oz.)	11–24
Lamb (3½ oz.)	100	Yogurt (½ cup)	8
Fish (3½ oz.)	50–60	Whipping cream, heavy (1 tbsp.)	20
Chicken (3½ oz.)	87	Cheese, Gouda (1 oz.)	21

*No more than 300 mg. cholesterol recommended per day

Why should a person limit salt intake?

Salt is the major source of the essential mineral sodium. In the days before refrigeration, people used salt to preserve foods; today salt is mainly a flavor enhancer. Unfortunately, sodium is related to high blood pressure, and it is not wise to rely on table salt for flavor. You could use a variety of herbs and spices instead. In addition, limit your intake of salty snack foods, and read food labels. Canned foods are generally high in sodium, and you should use them cautiously. The craving for salt is probably learned; to counteract it, most baby-food manufacturers have stopped adding salt to their products.

Why is sugar a problem?

Sugar is a simple carbohydrate that occurs naturally in grains, fruits, some vegetables, and milk; it is an important source of energy. The real culprit is the refined sugar used in soft drinks, candy, sweet desserts, and other processed food. The sugar problem results when "empty-calorie" foods replace the more nutrient-dense and naturally occurring carbohydrates you need. Excessive sugar intake also contributes to tooth decay and obesity.

Why should individuals limit caffeine intake?

Caffeine is a stimulant and thus the opposite of alcohol, a depressant. It is in coffee, colas and other soft drinks, tea, chocolate, and cocoa. This drug is often in candies and is combined in other drugs as well. Some of caffeine's many side effects include: frequent urination, sleeplessness, irregular heart beat, and extreme nervousness. If you like the taste of coffee and cola, try those that are caffeine free. If this doesn't work for you, limit the amount you consume.

Doing the java jive.

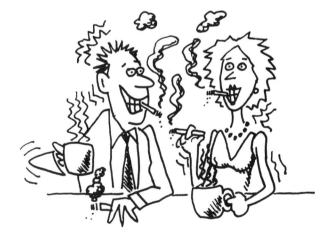

Is taking protein, vitamin, and mineral supplements necessary for exercising?

No. Unless you have specific symptoms of nutritional deficiency or unless you are certain that your dietary intake is inadequate, there should be no need for you to take any supplements at all. A balanced diet, one that provides a variety of foods from the four basic food groups, should be sufficient to meet your nutritional needs. If you wish to maintain your weight, however, you may have to increase your caloric intake once you start exercising regularly. Three foods each day from the meat group and three from the milk group should provide ample protein, even for a growing child. So pass up commercial protein supplements: They are unnecessary and costly.

The same advice holds for vitamins and minerals. There is no indication that exercise depletes a body's vitamin reserves. A varied selection from all the food groups provides sufficient vitamins for any normal person's needs. Although potassium and iron may, in some cases, be depleted by prolonged vigorous exercise, even they need not be replaced by using expensive commercial supplements. You can easily prevent the muscular weakness and fatigue associated with potassium or iron depletion. Just include plenty of vegetables, citrus fruits, and bananas in your daily diet to provide potassium, and include meat (particularly liver), fish, beans, green leafy vegetables, and dried fruits for iron.

Do protein, vitamin, and mineral supplements improve an athlete's performance?

No. Athletes are always searching for a magic substance that will enhance their powers, and businesses are always ready to profit from their quest. Despite the fact that there is no scientific evidence that the use of food supplements can improve athletic performance, many athletes—amateurs and professionals alike—are convinced that it can, and many "miraculous" formulations are on the market. The fact is that excessive amounts of niacin and vitamins A and D can be dangerous. The best nutritional aid to good health and athletic performance is a balanced diet.

Does caffeine help ward off exhaustion in prolonged endurance activity?

The caffeine in two cups of coffee, taken sixty minutes before exercising, may delay the onset of exhaustion during extended activity, but there are risks to weigh against this supposed benefit. Caffeine acts as a stimulant on the brain and by so doing may forestall the sensation of fatigue. It stimulates cardiac output and muscular activity in general, and thus may help your body work harder for a time. But it also stimulates the production of urine—causing discomfort and inconvenience during a long-distance run, for example.

What exactly is "carbohydrate loading"?

Carbohydrate loading is a complicated technique sometimes used by long-distance runners to provide maximum energy during competition. You begin about seven days or so before your event by exercising for a sixty-to-ninety-minute (or more) workout—almost to the point of exhaustion. This depletes your muscle glycogen stores. About three to four days before the competition, drastically increase your intake of carbohydrate—eating spaghetti, bread, potatoes, and the like. This results in high levels of muscle glycogen to sustain you through the latter part of the race, when fatigue usually sets in. In theory, and in carefully managed practice, carbohydrate loading leaves an athlete with very high levels of glycogen in the

---

SUGGESTIONS FOR EATING MORE FIBER

1. **Eat a balanced diet.** It is better to get your fiber from a variety of foods than from supplements. In this way you benefit from the nutrients in the foods themselves as well as from the fiber. Less processed foods are more desirable.

2. **Drink lots of water.** Without adequate liquids, fiber may work in reverse and actually slow or even block elimination.

3. **Avoid overcooking.** Whenever possible, eat your fruits and vegetables raw. Skins, including potato skins, are excellent sources of fiber. Boiling, peeling, and processing reduce usable fiber.

4. **Eat some fiber at each meal.** This may lessen the unpleasant effects and increase the benefits.

5. **Choose fiber-rich foods.** Use whole wheat bread instead of white bread, brown rice instead of white rice, buckwheat pancakes instead of those made with refined flour. Remember, too, that a baked potato, particularly if you eat the skin, is better than french fries.

---

muscles, which can be called upon to meet the extreme demands of *prolonged* endurance competition. For anything but marathon competition, evidence is lacking that carbohydrate loading is beneficial. Past practice included severely limiting carbohydrate intake during the heavy training session five to seven days before competition. This is no longer recommended.

Why is fiber so much in the news?

Fiber is the undigestible material found in plants. It is not a nutrient in the way that carbohydrates, proteins, fats, vitamins, and minerals are, but many experts believe that intake of high-fiber foods should be increased to between 25 and 40 grams a day. The exact amount for individuals may differ and you may need to experiment. In general fibers tend to produce larger and softer stools that move through the system more quickly. Increased consumption of fruits, vegetables, whole-grain products, and foods high in fiber accompanied by a low-fat diet may lower cholesterol and contribute to the prevention of colon cancer.

Studies have shown that oat bran, beans, and other foods high in soluble fiber may also increase the level of HDL, an important consideration in a heart healthy diet.

If you increase fiber intake too quickly, you may suffer some unpleasant side effects. These can include excessive intestinal gas, cramps, bloating, and even diarrhea. These usually diminish after a few days and may be avoided if fiber is added to your diet gradually via a variety of grains, fruits, and vegetables over a period of time. See "Suggestions for Eating More Fiber."

Is fish oil important in reducing the risk of heart disease?

There is some question as to whether fish oil supplements are of great value. What may be important is to increase the amount of cold-water fish in your diet. A

TABLE 6-7   Fat Content of Fish

The higher the fat the better the EPA (omega-3 fatty acids).

High Fat		Medium Fat	Low Fat	
salmon	shad	bass	cod	snapper
mackerel	sable	bluefish	flounder	brook trout
herring	most trout	carp	halibut	sea bass
sardines	mullet	catfish	haddock	sole
anchovies	bonito	whiting	perch	crappie
pompano	tuna*	sturgeon	pike	tilefish
whitefish		swordfish		

*Not canned in water
SOURCE: Adapted from *Runner's World,* Feb. '86.

twenty-year study of Dutch men found that those who ate the most fish suffered the lowest incidence of heart attack. The researchers suggested that one or two fish dishes per week on a regular basis may be of some health benefit. See Table 6-7, "Fat Content of Fish."

What is the best time to eat before an athletic event, and what should the meal consist of?

If you eat a meal about three hours before an athletic event, you allow enough time for the food to be digested and absorbed, but not enough time for you to feel hungry again. Many athletes still prefer a hearty steak-and-potatoes kind of meal, but most authorities now advise a menu designed to avoid discomfort and improve performance. Foods likely to cause discomfort include anything that is hard to digest, such as foods rich in fat. Avoid foods such as cabbage, beans, and cauliflower, which cause gas to build up in the intestine. Stay away from foods you are not used to eating. Avoid foods high in protein and cellulose—such as meat and leafy vegetables—which may increase your need to urinate or defecate during your activity period. Foods with some protein are recommended because some of the amino acids making up the proteins are converted to blood sugar by the liver. Spicy or salty food may make you thirsty and so should also be omitted.

Choose foods high in carbohydrate—spaghetti, bread, and potatoes—to give you quick energy without undue stress on the digestive system. Drink at least two or three glasses of fluid to be sure of adequate hydration. Table sugar or candy, though pure carbohydrate and regarded by many as a good source of instant energy, is of no proven value and may be detrimental. Excessive sugar may cause water retention in the digestive tract and thus interfere with the circulatory and heat regulatory systems so important in endurance exercise, especially in hot weather.

Is it wise to keep your weight down so you can compete in sports that are based on weight classifications?

No. For example, if muscular adolescents starve themselves to keep their weight down, their bodies are forced to obtain energy from muscle breakdown. The health risks connected with starvation or drying out in order to make the right weight classification (for a wrestling team, for instance) can be serious.

▇ Do alcohol and exercise mix?

Not very well. A small amount of alcohol—a glass of wine or beer at mealtime about three hours prior to exercise, say—is unlikely to have an adverse effect on activity. Larger amounts, however, can impair coordination or interfere with your exercise performance.

Alcohol is a central nervous system depressant that slows down the action of brain centers and reflex systems. The more you drink, the stronger the effects, although the effect of a given amount of alcohol may vary with such factors as your body size, prior use of alcohol, and how fast you down a drink. One or two drinks may slightly reduce motor efficiency, while three or four drinks can result in significant loss of coordination. It takes about one hour, on average, to metabolize one ounce of alcohol.

Contrary to folklore, drinking alcohol before exercising in cold weather will not really warm you up. When you take a drink, the blood circulation to your extremities increases. This may make your hands and feet feel warm at first, but it ultimately has a chilling effect, since the heat is easily lost from the extremities. The anesthetic effect of alcohol may also dull the skin's sensitivity to cold and thus deprive you of an important warning signal of overexposure to the cold. Lastly, the loss of judgment and locomotor control possible with heavy alcohol use poses significant dangers for people who engage in high-risk activities such as water sports, mountain climbing, skiing, and biking.

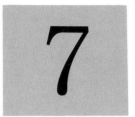

Model Exercise Programs

After you've read this chapter, you will be able to:

Differentiate among the purposes and procedures of the model programs.

Select and pursue one or more model programs consistent with your personal fitness goals.

By showing you how to get started and by setting reasonable standards for performance, a model program can launch you effectively into exercise and keep you going. It gives you a structured way to apply progressive overload and specificity—the two key training principles. If you stick with a model program, your fitness is bound to improve.

If you're fit enough to exercise, you're qualified to start a model program. None of them requires more than entry-level skills. You would not need any special sports ability or experience to begin a model program. Chances are you can find one in this chapter that demands little more in the way of athletic skills than those you have already.

CHOOSING A MODEL PROGRAM

Your task now is to select the appropriate program from among the eight basic models we present in this chapter. We have developed these models based on our experience designing regimens to meet almost every kind of fitness goal and to strengthen all of the fitness components. We have fully tested the eight prototypes presented, and they give realistic results.

Thus your challenge is not deciding whether a particular model program is likely to be effective, but rather deciding which one is going to be right for you. To choose a model program, begin by reviewing your specific fitness goals (see Table 1-2 in Chapter 1). That should be your starting point. Using Table 1-2, you can tie in your fitness goals to the fitness components involved in achieving them. Then turn to Table 7-1 to find out which model programs are likely to benefit the particular components you have to concentrate on to attain your fitness goals.

Next, narrow your choice. Read through the descriptions of the programs you're considering and decide which model will work best for you. Your final selection should be a program that adapts well to your present routine, seems enjoyable, and sounds like something you can start without major changes in your lifestyle. Avoid a time-consuming regimen if you're already overscheduled. Or if the early morning will be your time to exercise and you tend to wake up cranky and untalkative, stick to a simple program that you can follow in splendid isolation.

Agreed, no model program is likely to change you very much during the first few weeks of exercise. But what if the exercise program you chose does not seem suitable after you try it for a reasonable time? All may not be lost. It's possible that you can make adjustments in a model program to adapt it to your particular needs. But give the program a chance: Don't be too hasty about making changes. For three to four weeks, follow faithfully the specifics of the model program you chose. Then, if you do decide to adapt the regimen so it becomes more suited to your likes and dislikes, be sure you retain the basic elements of the program. For example, you may decide to change the specific exercises in the interval circuit training model program but keep the system intact. Don't change the amount of time specified for exercise or rest.

TABLE 7-1   Relating Model Programs to Fitness Components

For each model program listed below, a rating of high (H), moderate (M), or low (L) indicates the extent to which the program benefits each of the five components of physical fitness.

	Components of Physical Fitness				
Model program	Cardio-respiratory endurance	Body composition	Muscular strength*	Muscular endurance*	Flexibility*
Walking/jogging/running	H	H	M	H	L
Interval circuit training	H	H	H	H	M
Calisthenic circuit training	H	H	M	H	M
Stretching (warm-up/cool-down)	L	L	L	L	H
Bicycling	H	H	M	H	M
Rope skipping	H	H	M	H	L
Swimming	H	M	M	H	M
Weight training	L	M	H	H	H

*Ratings for these components are based on benefits for the specific muscle groups used during the activity in question. (See description of exercises for these model programs in this chapter to identify the muscle groups benefited.) For all other muscle groups, the rating would be low (L).

WALKING/JOGGING/RUNNING

Walking, jogging, and running are the most popular options for those who want to improve cardiorespiratory endurance (CRE) and body composition. Exercise on foot is by far the most common form of CRE training in the United States. These days there may be as many as 17 million people who jog regularly. And millions more walk as their favorite form of exercise. Walking, jogging, and running require no special skills, expensive equipment, or unusual facilities. Comfortable clothing, well-fitted walking or running shoes, and a stopwatch or ordinary watch with a second hand are all you need. What's more, like most CRE activities, they are effective techniques for weight control and changing body composition. They will also improve muscular endurance of the legs.

It's not always easy to distinguish among these three forms of CRE activities. Walking may vary from a 2-mile-per-hour pace that is leisurely for most people but may be taxing for others to a 9-mile-per-hour competitive pace that is faster than some can jog or run. When the pace is between 7 or 8 miles per hour, it's just as hard to tell where jogging ends and running begins. For clarity and consistency, we will consider *walking* any on-foot exercise of less than 5 miles per hour, *jogging* any pace between 5 and 7.5 miles per hour, and *running* any pace faster than that.

Table 7-2 divides walking, jogging, and running into nine categories with rates of speed and calorie costs for each. As you see, these activities can use a relatively large number of calories per minute. The faster your pace or the longer you exer-

---

TABLE 7-2   Walking/Jogging/Running

This table gives the calorie costs of walking, jogging, and running for a slow, moderate, and fast pace. Calculations for calorie costs are based on calories per minute per pound. They are approximate and assume a level terrain. A hilly terrain would result in higher calorie cost. Use this method to get an estimate of the number of calories you burn: Multiply your weight by the calories per minute per pound (listed in the right-hand column) for the speed at which you're doing the activity.

	Speed		
	---	---	---
Activity	Miles per hour	Minutes: seconds per mile	Calories per minute per pound
Walking			
Slow	2.0	30:00	.020
	2.5	24:00	.023
Moderate	3.0	20:00	.026
	3.5	17:08	.029
Fast	4.0	15:00	.037
	4.5	13:20	.048
Jogging			
Slow	5.0	12:00	.060
	5.5	11:00	.074
Moderate	6.0	10:00	.081
	6.7	9:00	.088
Fast	7.0	8:35	.092
	7.5	8:00	.099
Running			
Slow	8.5	7:00	.111
Moderate	9.0	6:40	.116
Fast	10.0	6:00	.129
	11.0	5:30	.141

cise, the more calories you burn. The greater the amount of calories burned, the higher the potential effectiveness of these activities for developing and maintaining CRE, improving body composition, and losing weight. Singly or in any combination, walking, jogging, or running can be done briskly enough to keep your heart rate within the exercise benefit zone (EBZ) long enough to burn a large number of calories each session. (See Chapter 3 for a discussion of EBZ.) By gradually increasing the total number of calories you use, you can progress to a level of fitness required to achieve your goals. Once you achieve the fitness level you set as your goal, you can occasionally ease up a bit on intensity and duration and reduce frequency.

The five variations of the basic walking/jogging/running model program that follow are designed to help you regulate the intensity, duration, and frequency of your program. To select the particular model that's best for you at your current CRE level, consult Table 7-3.

TABLE 7-3   Selecting a Walking/Jogging/Running Model Program

Model program 1: walking (starting)

Choose this program if *any* of the following apply:
   You have medical restrictions.
   You are recovering from illness or surgery.
   You tire easily after short walks.
   You are 50 pounds or more overweight.
   You have a sedentary lifestyle.
And if you want to prepare for the advanced walking program (see below) to improve CRE, body
   composition, and muscular endurance.

Model program 2: walking (advanced)

Choose this program if:
   You already can walk comfortably for 30 minutes.
And if you want to develop and maintain cardiorespiratory fitness, a lean body, and muscular
   endurance.

Model program 3: walking/jogging (starting)

Choose this program if:
   You already can walk comfortably for 30 minutes.
And if you want to prepare for the jogging/running program (see below) to improve CRE, body
   composition, and muscular endurance.

Model program 4: jogging/running

Choose this program if both of the following apply:
   You already can jog comfortably without muscular discomfort.
   You already can jog for 15 minutes within your EBZ without stopping or for 30 minutes with brief
      walking intervals.
And if you want to develop and maintain a high level of cardiorespiratory fitness, a lean body, and
   muscular endurance.

Model program 5: running (racing)

Choose this program if *all* the following apply:
   You already can jog/run comfortably within your EBZ for 30 to 60 minutes.
   You have been jogging/running regularly for at least 3 months.
   You have had a stress test (if you are among those for whom one is recommended—see pp. 4–5).
And if you want to train for road races as a way of maintaining a high level of cardiorespiratory fitness,
   a lean body, and muscular endurance.

General Guidelines for a Walking/Jogging/Running Program

Here are some guidelines to help you make whichever model program you select an effective training regimen. (Also see Chapter 12 for information on related matters.)

EBZ and Heart Rate   To measure progress with any of these model programs, you will need to know how to take your pulse (see p. 54) and how to determine your EBZ. All five walking/jogging/running model programs are based on raising heart rate into the EBZ. To work effectively for CRE training or to improve body composition, you may need to adjust your pace as you increase in fitness. Monitor your pulse to find out if your heart rate is in your EBZ.

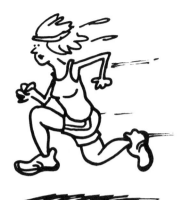

*It's not how fast you run that counts but how
well you keep your heart rate within your EBZ.*

Intensity   Begin *very* slowly if you're a novice at exercise or used to a sedentary lifestyle. Give your muscles a chance to adjust to the increased work load. At the outset, it may be wise to keep your heart rate below the EBZ until your body has had time to adapt to new demands.

  Even if you're not a beginner, you may find you're going at a slow pace because at first you may not need to walk or jog very fast to keep your heart rate in the EBZ. As your CRE improves, however, you will probably need to increase intensity. As you progress in CRE, chances are that you not only will pick up the pace automatically, but you may discover you don't even need to take your pulse to find out if your heart rate is in your EBZ. For one thing, if you exercise with a friend, you can rely on the "talk test"—the ability to keep up a conversation comfortably during exercise.

Duration and Frequency   To experience training effects, we recommend a minimum of fifteen minutes of exercise within the EBZ each session for model programs 2 through 5. Frequency of exercise should be three times a week—more often if your goal includes changing body composition or losing weight.

Interval Training   Some of the model programs involve continuous activity; others rely on interval training, which calls for alternating a relief interval with exercise (walking after you jog, say). Interval training can prolong the total time you spend in exercise and delay the onset of fatigue. A *set* is a combination of an exercise interval and a relief (or rest) interval.

Warm-Up and Cool-Down   No matter which one of the walking/jogging/running model programs you select, always begin each exercise session with a ten-minute warm-up. (See warm-up/cool-down in stretching model program.) This will help prevent loss of flexibility, which could be caused by the limited range of motion in walking/jogging/running. Avoid an abrupt transition from the warm-up phase to the active portion of your workout. To extend the warm-up period, begin your walk, jog, or run at a slower than usual pace to the point where you can maintain your workout within the EBZ. As you're ending your exercise session, always slow down gradually to bring your system back to its normal state. In addition to cooling down, it's a good idea to repeat the stretching exercises that were part of your warm-up.

Record-Keeping It's important to keep track of how you do on a walk/jog/run program. After each exercise session, record your daily distance (or time) on a progress chart set up to show your weekly totals (see Profile 13-3 in Chapter 13). At the end of each week, enter the total distance (or time) for the week and the total amount of calories expended in your exercise sessions.

Model Program 1: Walking (Starting)

Purpose To prepare for the advanced walking program to improve CRE, body composition, and muscular endurance.

Intensity Start at 50 to 60 percent of estimated maximum heart rate (MHR), which is below your EBZ. (See Chapter 3 for a discussion of how to calculate MHR and EBZ.) Gradually increase your pace, still keeping below your EBZ.

Duration Walk at first for fifteen minutes at a comfortable pace. Gradually increase to thirty-minute sessions. Distance will vary from one to two miles.

Frequency At the beginning, walk every other day. Gradually increase to daily walking if your purpose includes achieving a lean body.

Calorie Cost Work up to using about 90 to 135 calories in each session. (See Table 7-4.)

Progression Once your muscles have become adjusted to the exercise program, increase the duration of your sessions—but no more than 10 percent a week. Increase your intensity only enough to keep your heart rate just below your EBZ. When you're able to walk one and a half miles in thirty minutes, using from 90 to 135 calories per session, you should consider moving on to conditioning yourself to a maintenance walking program—model program 2: walking (advanced)—or to model program 3: walking/jogging (starting).

At the Beginning Start the walking model program at whatever level you feel comfortable. Maintain a normal easy pace and stop to rest as often as you need to.

Walk the routes you enjoy—and be on the lookout for pleasant new routes for walks.

From the beginning, try to walk every other day, even if the walk lasts only a few minutes. Never prolong a walk past the point of comfort. If you overdo, you're likely to end up with sore muscles and maybe even injuries—the path to becoming an "exercise drop-out."

Walking with a friend may help keep you going so try to persuade someone to join you. When walking with a friend, let a comfortable conversation be your guide to pace.

As You Progress Don't be discouraged by lack of immediate progress. And don't try to speed things up by overdoing, especially if your life has been sedentary. The change to a schedule of regular slow-paced walking will be sufficient to improve your CRE.

TABLE 7-4   Determining Calorie Cost Using Model Programs 1, 2, and 3

This table gives the approximate calorie costs per pound of body weight of walking or walking/jogging from 15 minutes to 60 minutes for distances of .50 mile up to 5.25 miles at varying rates of speed. These calorie costs are based on walking or jogging on a level terrain. To use the table, find on the horizontal line the approximate length of time you walk or jog. Then locate on the vertical column the approximate distance you cover. The figure at the intersection represents an estimate of the calories used per pound of body weight. Multiply this figure by your own body weight to get the total number of calories used. For example, assuming you weigh 135 pounds and walk 3.50 miles in 60 minutes, you would burn 235 calories: 1.74 (calories per pound, from table) × 135 (weight) = 235 calories.

Distance (in miles)	Time (in minutes)									
	15	20	25	30	35	40	45	50	55	60
.50	.30									
.75	.39	.43	.47							
1.00	.56	.52	.56	.60						
1.25	.90	.63	.65	.69						
1.50	1.20	.96	.74	.78	.82					
1.75	1.39	1.32	1.03	.87	.91	.95	.99			
2.00		1.61	1.38	1.11	1.00	1.04	1.08	1.12		
2.25		1.79	1.78	1.44	1.18	1.13	1.17	1.21	1.25	1.29
2.50			2.01	1.81	1.47	1.27	1.26	1.30	1.34	1.38
2.75			2.19	2.23	1.85	1.57	1.35	1.39	1.43	1.47
3.00			2.37	2.41	2.22	1.92	1.67	1.48	1.52	1.56
3.25				2.59	2.63	2.23	1.96	1.76	1.61	1.65
3.50					2.81	2.65	2.29	2.06	1.83	1.74
3.75						3.03	2.71	2.39	2.08	1.90
4.00						3.21	3.10	2.76	2.41	2.23
4.25							3.43	3.15	2.78	2.50
4.50							3.61	3.57	3.18	2.87
4.75								3.83	3.51	3.19
5.00								4.01	3.96	3.62
5.25									4.23	3.97

Soon you may be walking for a longer time than usual and taking fewer and shorter rest stops. You may feel instinctively when it would be comfortable to pick up the pace. As you approach your target of a comfortable thirty-minute walk, you may be able to increase your rate of speed enough so that you approach the lower level of your EBZ (70 percent of your MHR). The pace at which different people walk in order to reach 70 percent of estimated MHR can vary considerably. For some, it will be a slow 2 miles per hour. For others, it will be a moderate 3.5 miles per hour. Of course, pace and heart rate can vary with the terrain, the weather, and other factors.

Measuring Calories   Suppose you begin this model program with a fifteen-minute walk for one-half mile. A look at Table 7-4 will show that if you weigh 154 pounds you would have burned 46 calories. If you walk double the distance in just a few more minutes, you will almost double the number of calories you use. But the rate of speed would also have to double, and that pace may be too taxing for anyone whose beginning CRE dictated selection of this model program. Instead, you should aim to increase calorie costs by walking for a longer time or for a longer distance rather than by increasing your rate of speed.

Model Program 2: Walking (Advanced)

Purpose   To develop and maintain cardiorespiratory fitness, a lean body, and muscular endurance.

Intensity   Start at a pace within your EBZ but soon begin to walk at a little faster pace. This might boost your heart rate into the upper levels of your EBZ, which is fine for brief periods. But don't overdo the intervals of fast walking. Slow down after a short time to drop your pulse rate. Gradually, you can lengthen the periods of fast walking and shorten the relief intervals of slow walking. Vary your regimen to allow for intervals of slow, medium, and fast walking.

Duration   Walk at first for thirty minutes. Gradually increase your walking time until eventually you reach sixty minutes, all the while keeping within your EBZ. Distance will vary from two to four miles.

Frequency   Walk every other day. Exercise more frequently if your purpose includes changing body composition.

Calorie Cost   Work up to using about 200 to 350 calories in each session. (See Table 7-4.)

Progression   As your heart rate adjusts to the increased work load, gradually increase your pace and your total walking time. Interval training is an effective way to achieve progressive overload: When your heart rate gets too high, slow down to lower your pulse rate until you're at the low end of your EBZ. Eventually, you will reach the fitness level you would like to maintain. For some, it may be the ability to walk at a rapid 4 miles per hour for thirty minutes; for others, it may be a more leisurely walk extending over sixty minutes or longer. To maintain the level of fitness you choose for yourself, continue to burn the same amount of calories as you did to reach that fitness level.

At the Beginning   Begin the advanced walking program by keeping within your familiar thirty-minute walking time but walk somewhat faster. Check your pulse to make sure you keep your heart rate within your EBZ. Slow down when necessary to lower your heart rate when going up hills or when extending the duration of your walks. Using this form of interval training, you will gradually be able to extend the periods of faster walking and decrease the number and length of the relief intervals of slow walking. In time, you will be able to walk for longer than thirty minutes and at a faster pace as your CRE level improves, with your heart rate remaining comfortably within your EBZ.

Sonia decided that for her busy schedule at school, brisk walking would be the way to get and stay in shape. She started with a daily mile and gradually worked up to four miles. Once she reached 4 miles per hour at a moderate-to-fast pace, she was able to maintain her fitness level even though she skipped a day or two or cut back from a walk of four miles to three.

At her low weight of 98 pounds, Sonia uses about 219 calories during each sixty-minute session. In a typical week of daily walking, she does more than 1,500 calories' worth of exercise, a total that apparently played a part in altering her body composition. Sonia has lost one to two inches each from her waist, hips, and thighs and is maintaining her 5-foot frame in this condition. Sonia credits her regular walking program with helping her to eliminate midafternoon fatigue and sleep well at night. What's more, Sonia says, "My walk is my thinking/problem-solving time."

As You Progress   Vary your regimen by changing the pace and distance walked or by walking routes with different terrains and views. Some days, too, you might have only limited time for exercise. If your usual workout consists of a leisurely 3-mile-per-hour walk that takes sixty minutes, try the following variations if you need to save time and still keep your exercise schedule: Increase your intensity to as much as 4.5 miles per hour and decrease your duration and distance by walking two and a quarter miles in thirty minutes. Don't use this option, however, if by speeding up your pace you move your heart rate beyond your EBZ for longer than brief periods.

As you progress, maintain your heart rate within your EBZ. Do not, as a regular practice, keep your pulse high for more than brief periods. Although picking up the pace can burn more calories per minute, it also promotes fatigue—thus tending to limit the duration of the session. In the end, you could be burning fewer calories. Make use of interval training with its regulated control of pace to maintain your heart rate at a desired level. It also introduces variety into a continuous walking program done at the same pace—a monotonous prospect for some.

Measuring Calories   Table 7-4 will help you assess the calorie benefits of time spent doing model program 2. Use the table to give direction to your sessions and to gauge progress toward whatever calorie goal you've set.

Model Program 3: Walking/Jogging (Starting)

Purpose   To prepare for the jogging/running program to improve CRE, body composition, and muscular endurance.

Intensity   Start by walking at a moderate pace (3 to 4 miles per hour). Staying within your EBZ, begin to add brief intervals of slow jogging (5 to 6 miles per hour). Keep the walking intervals constant at sixty seconds or at 110 yards. Gradually increase the jogging intervals.

Duration   Each exercise session should last fifteen to thirty minutes, alternating walking with jogging. Eventually, your time spent jogging will be at least four times as long as for walking. Distances will vary from one and a half to two and a half miles.

Frequency   Exercise every other day. Exercise more frequently by walking only, on days you're not walking/jogging, if your purpose includes changing body composition.

TABLE 7-5   Sample Walking/Jogging Progression by Time

This table is based on a walking interval of 3.75 miles per hour, measured in seconds, and a jogging interval of 5.5 miles per hour, measured in minutes: seconds. The combination of the two intervals equals a single set. Under the heading "Number of sets," the higher figure represents the maximum number of sets to be completed.

Walk interval (seconds)	Jog interval (minutes: seconds)	Number of sets	Total distance (miles)	Total time (minutes: seconds)
:60	:30	10–15	1.0–1.7	15:00–22:30
:60	:60	8–13	1.2–2.0	16:00–26:00
:60	2:00	5–19	1.3–2.3	15:00–27:00
:60	3:00	5–7	1.6–2.4	16:00–28:00
:60	4:00	3–6	1.5–2.7	15:00–30:00

TABLE 7-6   Sample Walking/Jogging Progression by Distance

This table is based on a walking interval of 3.75 miles per hour, measured in yards, and a jogging interval of 5.5 miles per hour, also measured in yards. The combination of the two intervals equals a single set.

Walk interval (yards)	Jog interval (yards)	Number of sets	Total distance (miles)	Total time (minutes: seconds)
110	55	11–21	1.0–2.0	15:00–28:12
110	110	16	2.0	26:56
110	220	11	2.0	26:02
110	330	8	2.0	24:24
110	440	7	2.2	26:05
110	440	8	2.5	29:49

Calorie Cost   Work up to using about 200 to 350 calories in each session. (See Table 7-4.)

Progression   Choose the walking/jogging progression that suits you best—one based on either time (see Table 7-5) or distance (see Table 7-6). Adjust your ratio of walking to jogging, as you increase your jogging, to keep within your EBZ as much as possible. When you have progressed to the point where most of your thirty-minute session is spent jogging, you should consider moving on to model program 4: jogging/running.

Even after you move on to model program 4, you will find it useful to go back to walking/jogging, perhaps combined with features of the jogging/running program, as an effective way to maintain high levels of fitness.

At the Beginning   Start the walking/jogging program slowly. Until your muscles adjust to jogging, you may need to exercise at less than your EBZ. At the outset, expect to do two to four times as much walking as jogging. If you're relatively inexperienced at jogging and find your heart rate is consistently at the top of your EBZ or above it, you may need to do even more walking than that. Be guided by how comfortable you feel—and by your heart rate—in setting the pace for your progress. At first, check your heart rate often. In time you should develop a sense of when you're in your EBZ. But don't overdo: Limit your progress to weekly increments of not more than 10 percent in intensity or duration.

Lorraine began a walk/jog program at her physician's suggestion. She described herself to Consumers Union as having become "rather flabby and generally out of shape" with various medical problems. Already accustomed to walking extensively, Lorraine took a stress test before beginning a jogging program "to be on the safe side." Her program consisted of eight weeks of brisk walking for at least thirty minutes (or one and a half to two miles) three to four times a week. In the second eight weeks, Lorraine began jogging on a two-to-one ratio (two parts walk to one part jog). She confesses to having been "a total flop" at taking her pulse as she increased the level of exercise because she never learned to "distinguish between the beat of my pulse and the noises around me."

Lorraine's exercise regimen and a careful diet combined to do away with "most of the flab" (17 pounds' worth). Running on city sidewalks, however, contributed to "painful knee problems" as did, perhaps, a tendency on Lorraine's part to give short shrift to her stretching exercises.

As You Progress   Like Lorraine, once she phased into jogging, you may have started on a two-to-one ratio. Assume your plan is to progress to a one-to-four ratio—one part walk to four parts jog. (The number of sets—the combinations of exercise and relief intervals—that you do in an exercise session may range from three to twenty-one.) To make it easier to organize your workouts and to measure progress, keep the walking interval constant at sixty seconds or 110 yards as you gradually increase the jogging interval. You may complete anywhere from one mile to more than two and a half miles within fifteen to thirty minutes.

To find a walking/jogging progression that suits you, refer to Tables 7-5 and 7-6. (One uses time, the other distance.) Which one you choose will depend, to some extent, on where you work out. If you have access to a track or can use a measured distance with easily visible landmarks to indicate yardage covered, you may find it convenient to use distance as your organizing principle. If you'll be using parks, streets, or woods, time intervals (measured with a watch) would probably work better.

The suggested progressions in Tables 7-5 and 7-6—by time or distance—are not meant to be rigid mandates. Rather, they embody guidelines to help you develop your own rate of progress. The tables are based on a pace of 3.75 miles per hour for walking and of 5.5 miles per hour for jogging, but don't be bound by that: Adjust your tempo to what suits you best. For some people, the recommended beginning two-to-one ratio or the suggested rate of speed may be too low or too high. No matter which method you follow, let your progress be guided by your heart rate. Increase intensity and duration only to get your heart rate into the EBZ.

Measuring Calories   Table 7-4 will help you assess the calorie benefits of the time you spend doing model program 3. Use this table to guide and measure your progress toward an energy expenditure of 200 to 350 calories each session. Walking and jogging for thirty minutes, covering about one and a half to two and a half miles, will cause a typical exerciser to burn about 200 to 350 calories each exercise session, totaling about 600 to 1,050 calories a week with three workouts a week. For a person with low to moderate CRE levels, the calorie cost—if expended by working within the EBZ—is enough to guarantee progress in improving CRE fitness.

Model Program 4: Jogging/Running

Purpose   To develop and maintain a high level of cardiorespiratory fitness, a lean body, and muscular endurance.

Intensity   The key is to keep within your EBZ. Most people who sustain a continuous jog/run program will find that they can stay within their EBZ at a rate of speed between 5.5 and 7.5 miles per hour. Find out for yourself what intensity keeps you in your EBZ.

Duration   Start by jogging steadily for fifteen minutes. Gradually increase your jog/run session to a regular thirty to sixty minutes (or about two and a half to seven miles).

Frequency   Exercise every other day. Exercise more frequently—but alternate with other activities (see below)—if your purpose includes achieving a lean body.

Calorie Cost   Use about 300 to 750 calories in each session. (See Table 7-7.)

Progression   If you chose model program 4, you probably already have moderate to high CRE. To improve CRE further, increase your distance or both pace and distance to burn additional calories. But make these adjustments only if you need to get your heart rate into the EBZ.

At the Beginning   When you start this program, you already can jog comfortably for fifteen minutes without any muscular discomfort. But with this program you will be gradually increasing the time you spend jogging and doing it in a way that prevents muscle and joint problems. Be consistent about your warm-up stretching. Do not make the commitment to this model program if you're likely to skimp on time for warm-up and cool-down.

If one of your purposes in exercising is to achieve a lean body, and if your exercise time is limited, model program 4 can make an effective contribution. The greater number of calories you burn per minute (see Table 7-7) makes this regimen less time-consuming for altering body composition and losing weight than the three previous programs in the walking/jogging/running series.

Even if you have ample time for daily exercise, you still may wish to use model program 4. If your purpose is to lose weight or change body composition, it isn't necessary to use the model every day. Instead, on alternate days do long-distance walking (see model program 2) or some other high-calorie activity such as swimming or bicycling. Increasing frequency by using these supplemental activities will place less stress on the weight-bearing parts of the lower body than a daily regimen of jogging/running.

TABLE 7-7   Determining Calorie Cost Using Model Program 4

This table gives the approximate calorie costs of a jogging/running program from 15 to 60 minutes for distances from 1.25 to 8 miles at varying rates of speed on a level terrain. (For a slower pace, refer to Table 7-4.) To use the table, find on the horizontal line the approximate length of time you jog/run. Then locate on the vertical column the approximate distance you cover. The figure at the intersection represents an estimate of the calories used per pound of body weight. Multiply this figure by your own body weight to get the total number of calories used. For example, assuming you weigh 135 pounds and jog 3 miles in 30 minutes, you would burn 325 calories: 2.41 (calories per pound, from table) × 135 (weight) = 325 calories.

Distance (in miles)	Time (in minutes)									
	15	20	25	30	35	40	45	50	55	60
1.25	.90									
1.50	1.20									
1.75	1.39									
2.00	1.57	1.61								
2.25	1.75	1.79								
2.50	1.93	1.97	2.01							
2.75		2.15	2.19	2.23						
3.00		2.33	2.37	2.41						
3.25		2.51	2.55	2.59	2.63					
3.50			2.73	2.77	2.81					
3.75			2.91	2.95	2.99	3.03				
4.00			3.09	3.13	3.17	3.21				
4.25				3.31	3.35	3.39	3.43			
4.50				3.49	3.53	3.57	3.61			
4.75					3.72	3.75	3.79	3.83		
5.00					3.90	3.94	3.98	4.01		
5.25					4.08	4.12	4.16	4.20	4.23	
5.50						4.30	4.34	4.38	4.42	4.46
5.75						4.48	4.52	4.56	4.60	4.64
6.00							4.70	4.74	4.78	4.82
6.25							4.88	4.92	4.96	5.00
6.50								5.10	5.14	5.18
6.75								5.28	5.32	5.36
7.00									5.50	5.54
7.25									5.68	5.72
7.50									5.86	5.90
7.75										6.08
8.00										6.27

Kyle, a college senior, told Consumers Union that he began jogging in a freshman conditioning class. After the first two weeks, he was able to jog a mile. By the end of the semester, he was able to jog three miles at 8 to 9 minutes per mile. After three years of continued jogging, Kyle covers five miles three or four times a week at a 7-minute-per-mile pace and feels that if he wanted to, he could go faster; however, he tries to keep his goals clear and resists the temptation to run too fast.

As You Progress   With a conditioning and maintenance program, it sometimes becomes necessary to forestall boredom. You can ease the monotony of the routine by varying the route, the intensity, and the duration. You may want to alternate short runs with long ones. If you run for sixty minutes one day, try running for thirty minutes for your next exercise session. Or try doing sets that alternate hard and easy intervals—even walking, if you feel like it. You could also try a road race now and then, but be careful not to do too much too soon. Many joggers listen to music to forestall boredom.

Variety and music can hold off boredom in your routine.

Measuring Calories   Table 7-7 will help you assess the calorie benefits of time spent doing model program 4. Use the table to guide and measure your progress toward burning the recommended 300 to 750 calories in each session.

Model Program 5: Running (Racing)

Purpose   To train for road races as a way of maintaining a high level of cardiorespiratory fitness, a lean body, and muscular endurance. A sample four-week program to train you for a first race of up to five miles is shown in Table 7-8.

Intensity   Once again, it is important to stay within your EBZ. In a road race, you should aim to complete the distance at a pace roughly equal to the one you use in your regular workouts. If you find a need to increase your work load, observe the 10 percent rule: no more than a 10 percent increase in intensity or duration each week.

Duration   Your workouts should range from thirty to sixty minutes of running within your EBZ. For your first race, find a "fun run"* that covers no more than three to five miles. Only after several of these should you try races over longer distances.

Frequency   Keep your participation in road racing to less than once a month. Frequency of workouts should be every other day. If you want to exercise more often, add other activities (see model program 4) on alternate days.

Calorie Cost   Use about 300 to 750 calories in each session.

Progression   Racing is not for everyone. But if you're a runner who enjoys competition and if you have the self-discipline to stick with a sensible rate of progress, road racing (or fun runs) can motivate you to achieve high levels of CRE. Training for road racing can be kept interesting and exciting: Add diversity to your sessions by using the different training techniques described below.

At the Beginning   Try to finish your first race while running at your usual workout pace. You may finish at the back of the pack, but that's fine if that's where your correct fitness level places you. While racing, don't be seduced by the excitement of

---

*"Fun runs" are local runs over measured distances. The emphasis is on one's personal accomplishment rather than on competition against others.

TABLE 7-8   Training Program for 5-Mile Road Race

The table below outlines a sample four-week program for preparing for a first road race of five miles or less. It uses long slow distance (LSD), interval training, and *fartlek* (see pp. 122–123) to illustrate how these techniques can be combined effectively. Of course, a regimen can be based on just one of the three, but the combination provides a more diversified and perhaps more interesting approach to training.* The regimen calls for stretching exercises on most alternate days. See stretching model program.

Week 1

Day 1   Run 30 to 60 minutes of LSD at a pace within your EBZ.
Day 2   Do stretching exercises.
Day 3   Do 30 to 60 minutes of *fartlek* on varied terrain at varied pace. Try to maintain your heart rate in your EBZ, but don't worry if your running segments bring your heart rate above your EBZ now and then. If done for an extended period, however, this can limit the duration of the session.
Day 4   Do stretching exercises.
Day 5   Run 30 to 60 minutes of LSD at a pace in the low to midrange of your EBZ.
Day 6   Do interval training. Run 440 yards at your time-goal pace (see Table 7-9, p. 123), then walk 30 to 90 seconds. Repeat the set 16 times. The length of the walk interval depends on how long it takes to bring your heart rate below your EBZ.
Day 7   Do stretching exercises.

Week 2

Day 1   Run 30 to 60 minutes of LSD at a pace in the low to midrange of your EBZ.
Day 2   Do stretching exercises.
Day 3   Do 30 to 60 minutes of *fartlek*.
Day 4   Do stretching exercises.
Day 5   Run 30 to 60 minutes of LSD within your EBZ.
Day 6   Do interval training. Run 880 yards at your time-goal pace, then walk 60 to 90 seconds. Repeat the set 10 times.
Day 7   Do stretching exercises.

Week 3

Day 1   Run 30 to 60 minutes of LSD at a pace within your EBZ.
Day 2   Do stretching exercises.
Day 3   Do 30 to 60 minutes of *fartlek*.
Day 4   Do stretching exercises.
Day 5   Run 30 to 60 minutes of LSD within your EBZ.
Day 6   Do interval training. Run 1 mile at your time-goal pace, then walk 220 yards, and jog 220 yards at a slow pace. Repeat the set 5 times.
Day 7   Do stretching exercises.

Week 4 (race week)

Day 1   Run 30 to 60 minutes of LSD at a pace within your EBZ.
Day 2   Do stretching exercises.
Day 3   Do interval training. Run 440 yards at your time-goal pace, then jog 220 yards at a slow pace. Repeat the set 16 times.
Day 4   Do stretching exercises.
Day 5   Run 30 minutes of LSD at a pace within your EBZ.
Day 6   Do stretching exercises.
Day 7   Run 5-mile race.

*Interval training complicates calorie calculation. A record of total time and distance covered will give you only a general indication of calories used. To get an idea of calorie cost, see Table 7-7.

competition. The surge of the crowd at the start, the tendency to set a fast pace, the adrenaline flowing freely, and sometimes an overwhelming desire to be a winner can trap you into running faster than you need to in order to stay within your EBZ. You're participating in regularly scheduled road races to help you stick with a regimen that will keep your CRE levels high and your body lean but not necessarily to win the races.

By the time most runners take part in road races, they can tell when they're within their EBZ without having to take their pulse constantly. Should you need to check your EBZ, find another runner to chat with during the race and rely on the talk test to adjust your pace.

Space your races to less than one a month: give yourself ample time to recover. And listen to your body. Each person is different in this regard. If you sense that you don't feel right in a race, avoid the tendency to "gut" it out. It's no disgrace to stop or slow down. If you feel like it, walk up a hill or stop for a drink of water. Hot days in particular can be a problem. (See Chapter 12 for more about running in hot weather.)

Neil, a 50-year-old schoolteacher, described for Consumers Union the culmination of his year-long progression from jogging to regular road racing. "Last Saturday I entered a 5-kilometer (3.1-mile) race. I came in second in my age group (over 50) with a time of 26:16. The winning time was run by a doctor—19:45. This was only the third race I had entered, and I finished second. What more motivation does a young man of 50 need?" During his years of jogging/running, Neil reports losing fifteen pounds, and his double chin and pot belly "are almost gone."

As You Progress   The key is slow steady progress: Increase mileage and pace by no more than 10 percent a week. You may not win the races you enter, but you're more likely to be free of injuries. At your own rate of progress, your satisfaction will come from setting occasional personal records—improving your time, adding to your distance, or moving up in the order of finish.

For many runners, a marathon seems the ultimate achievement. If you want to run in a marathon, be sure to progress slowly. Only after you have gradually and systematically worked up to longer distances should you set yourself such a challenge.

Marathoners and beginning road racers alike benefit from many of the same training techniques. When training for a race, there are several ways to add variety to your regimen.

Long Slow Distance (LSD)   This technique—running at a comfortable level within the EBZ for prolonged durations—is the foundation of your running program. LSD should also be the mainstay of your preparation for racing. Increase the length of your runs: If you stay within your EBZ, your CRE will improve and your intensity will automatically increase without conscious effort. Forget about dramatic efforts to make your super-racer fantasies come true: They may lead to injuries and spoil a good fitness program. If on occasion you want to run faster, try interval training or *fartlek* (see below).

Interval Training   By scheduling a resting interval alternately with a running interval—each combination is one set—interval training lets you extend a workout over a

TABLE 7-9   Walking/Jogging/Running Pace Chart

This table provides approximate times for distances from 110 yards to 5 miles and for rates of speed from 3 to 11 miles per hour. Use this table to set your time goals for interval training.

	Miles per hour	Distances (in hours:minutes:seconds)					
		5 miles	1 mile	880 yds. (½ mile)	440 yds. (¼ mile)	220 yds.	110 yds.
Walking							
Moderate	3.0	1:40:00	20:00	10:00	5:00	2:30	1:15
	3.75	1:20:00	16:00	8:00	4:00	2:00	1:00
Fast	4.5	1:07:45	13:33	6:46	3:23	1:41	:50
Jogging							
Slow	5.0	60:00	12:00	6:00	3:00	1:30	:45
	5.5	55:00	11:00	5:30	2:45	1:23	:41
Moderate	6.0	50:00	10:00	5:00	2:30	1:15	:37
	6.7	45:00	9:00	4:30	2:15	1:08	:34
Fast	7.0	42:55	8:35	4:18	2:09	1:04	:32
	7.5	40:00	8:00	4:00	2:00	1:00	:30
Running							
Slow	8.6	35:00	7:00	3:30	1:45	:53	:26
Moderate	9.0	33:20	6:40	3:20	1:40	:50	:25
Fast	10.0	30:00	6:00	3:00	1:30	:45	:22
	11.0	27:30	5:30	2:45	1:23	:41	:20

longer time. This technique delays the onset of fatigue. Suppose you want to prepare for a five-mile race that you hope to run in forty minutes—a pace of eight minutes per mile. You would then plan to run ten or more half-mile intervals at your pace or better (see Table 7-8). For resting intervals, you would walk or jog for up to ninety seconds or until your EBZ dips below minimum threshold levels.

With interval training, you can vary the distance and pace of the running period and the number of sets you do. The number and length of your resting intervals affect the intensity of the workout, as does the pace at which you run. Keep your workout interval below the upper level of your EBZ. Although there's no harm in a well-conditioned runner exceeding the EBZ now and then, overdoing it results in fatigue and limits the duration of the workout. See Table 7-9 for suggestions on pace.

Fartlek   Fartlek is Swedish for "play of speed." It's a training technique you can use when you want a change of pace from LSD. Just as LSD is steady and sensible, fartlek is freewheeling and unpredictable. With this technique, you can run as fast or slow as you like for as long or short a period as you choose, mixing sprints and walking in a long, unplanned, untimed, cross-country run in the woods, on beaches, up and down hills, or in any setting that provides a pleasant change of pace. The short bursts of speed can be exhilarating after a period on LSD training and the lack of structure can be welcome after interval training.

INTERVAL CIRCUIT TRAINING

Interval circuit training is a series of exercises, performed in sequence, and using several pieces of equipment (see below). This model program of nine exercises provides a workout for all major muscle groups and has the potential of improving CRE,

---

TABLE 7-10   Sample Log for Interval Circuit Training Program

In this sample progress chart for interval circuit training, the first column shows the exercises in the order they should be performed. The figures in the second column (1, 2, 3) represent the first, second, and third times around the circuit. In the other columns, enter the number of repetitions performed for the exercises each time you make your way around the circuit. As a guide, we have filled in the number of repetitions for what could be one day in each of your first three weeks on the model program. First week: once around the circuit on three alternate days. Second week: two consecutive turns around the circuit on three alternate days. Third week and weeks following: three consecutive turns around the circuit on three alternate days. When you want to add weight (+ wt.) to your equipment, you can record it as shown below.

Exercise		First week	Second week	Third week			
1. Bent rowing	1.	20	20	20 + wt.			
	2.		21	16			
	3.			18			
2. Sit-up	1.	18	19	18			
	2.		17	16			
	3.			17			
3. Clean and press	1.	17	17	18			
	2.		18	16			
	3.			18			
4. Curl	1.	25	26 + wt.	24			
	2.		26	25			
	3.			24			
5. Twister	1.	45	50	45			
	2.		48	40			
	3.			40			
6. Forward raise	1.	18	20	19			
	2.		19	16			
	3.			18			
7. Step-up	1.	20	19	19			
	2.		20	17			
	3.			19			
8. Push-up	1.	13	12	14			
	2.		10	12			
	3.			12			
9. Rope skipping	1.	25	35	35			
	2.		31	30			
	3.			35			

muscular strength, and muscular endurance. With this program, you can burn about 10 calories per minute.

In interval circuit training, each exercise should be performed at your maximum effort for thirty seconds, followed by fifteen seconds in which you record the number of repetitions performed and prepare for the next exercise. (See Table 7-10 for a sample progress chart.)

Interval Circuit Training Progress Card

Name _____

Exercise		First week	Second week	Third week			
1. Bent rowing	1. 2. 3.						
2. Sit-up	1. 2. 3.						
3. Clean and press	1. 2. 3.						
4. Curl	1. 2. 3.						
5. Twister	1. 2. 3.						
6. Forward raise	1. 2. 3.						
7. Step-up	1. 2. 3.						
8. Push-up	1. 2. 3.						
9. Rope skipping	1. 2. 3.						

Terminology

To use interval circuit training, you have to learn the language—some of which may be new to you.

Circuit Training   A system of organizing a series of exercises arranged for consecutive performance. In this program, nine exercises is one circuit.

Repetitions   The number of times you perform an exercise.

Exercise Interval   The time in which you perform an exercise at your maximum effort. For this program, thirty seconds is the exercise interval.

Rest Interval   The time following the performance of an exercise used to record the number of repetitions completed and to prepare for the next exercise. For this program, fifteen seconds is the rest interval.

Interval Circuit Training Program

Purpose   To develop and maintain all fitness components, primarily CRE and muscular endurance.

Equipment   One barbell, one swingbell (dumbbell bar with plates clamped in the center of the bar), slant board, bench or chair, jump rope, wand (broomsticklike length of wood doweling), cassette, and player (or large-faced clock with sweep-second hand).

Intensity   Because this model program is designed for muscular endurance, you'll exercise against low resistance with many repetitions. Because you exercise at high intensity (performing at maximum effort, i.e., as many repetitions as you can within a limited time), there is a fifteen-second rest interval between the performance of each exercise. The exercises are arranged so that the same muscle groups are not used in successive exercises, thus avoiding overtiring them.

Heart rates have been recorded at high levels during the performance of this model program. So monitor your pulse periodically and raise or lower the intensity (number of repetitions) to keep your heart rate within your exercise benefit zone.

Duration   Do three trips around the circuit, which should take about twenty minutes. That's enough to influence CRE. One or two circuits take less time and can be effective in developing muscular endurance. But fewer than three circuits would be of limited significance in improving CRE.

Frequency   Exercise three days per week.

At the Beginning

At a local fitness center or store that carries weight training equipment, experiment with a barbell until you find a weight you can use for at least 15 repetitions without strain.

After you have assembled all your equipment, set it up in your workout area so you can perform each exercise in the thirty seconds allowed. Read the instructions carefully on how to perform the exercises.

Always warm up. Do the stretching model program before you start your exercise period. To prevent excessive soreness, limit yourself to just one full circuit for the first three exercise periods. Go on to two full circuits for the next three exercise periods. From then on, each exercise period should consist of three complete circuits. A cassette can help you control your time around the circuit. Using a stopwatch, record your own voice saying: "Ready, begin. . . . Record and change," etc., allowing thirty seconds for the exercise interval followed by fifteen seconds for the rest interval.

Exercises for Interval Circuit Training Program

For best results, do the exercises in the numerical sequence below. It's important to perform at your maximum effort for the thirty-second exercise interval (followed by the fifteen-second rest interval in which to record and change). Doing the circuit as a whole will improve CRE. The body parts affected by the exercises are noted, as well as which exercises are especially useful for CRE.

1. **Bent rowing: barbell** (upper back, arms)
   With your back flat and knees bent, raise the barbell to your chest, keeping your elbows high.
   Safety: Do this exercise while resting your head on a table.

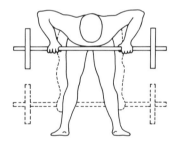

2. **Sit-up: slant board** (abdominals)
   If you use a slant board and can't do even one sit-up, start with your head at the high end of the board. As the sit-ups become easier, gradually lower the head of the board until you are doing sit-ups on a level surface. You can increase resistance by doing your sit-ups with your head at the lower end of the slant board. Always perform these exercises with your knees bent.

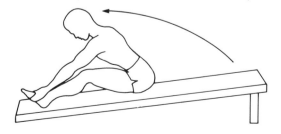 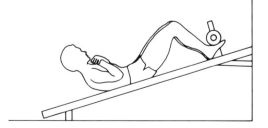

3. **Clean and press: barbell** (full body)

Lift the barbell from the floor to your chest in one movement and then push it over your head, using only your arms.

Safety: Be sure your knees are bent and your back is flat when lifting the barbell from the floor. Lifting is done with the legs, *not* with the back.

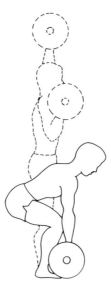

4. **Curl: barbell** (biceps, forearms)

With your palms forward and elbows close to your sides, bend your elbows, bringing the barbell up to your chest. Do not swing your body forward and back. Maintain a stationary position.

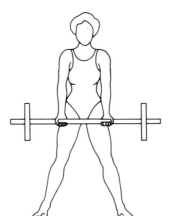 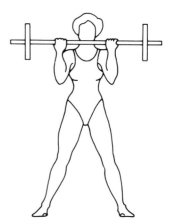

5. **Twister: wand** (hamstrings, trunk)
   Bend forward with your back flat, your head up, and your knees slightly bent. Twist your body to the left and then to the right. Touch first one foot and then the other. Keep your upper arm straight and over your back. (This can also be done with a wand or broomstick held across your shoulders.)

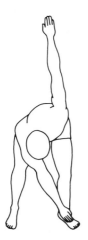 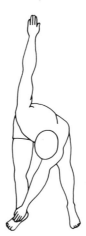

6. **Forward raise: dumbbells** (shoulders, upper back)
   With knuckles forward and your arms straight, raise both arms overhead and return to the starting position.

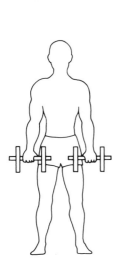 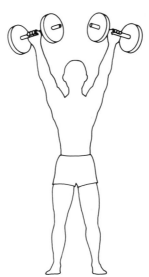

7. **Step-up: bench or chair** (thighs, hips, CRE)
Step up with first one foot and then the other, alternating rhythmically up and down. As one foot goes up, the other comes down. Individuals with pain underneath or around their knee caps should avoid this exercise.

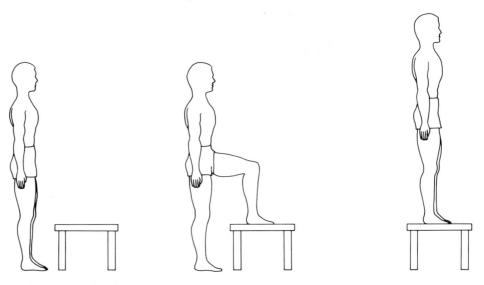

8. **Push-up** (chest, triceps, upper back)
Keeping your back and legs straight, push your body away from the floor. To add resistance, raise your feet and then lower your chest to the floor.

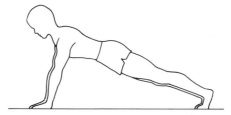

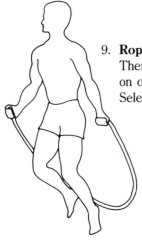

9. **Rope skipping: rope** (CRE, legs)
There are many ways to skip rope, but the most common techniques are jumping on one foot at a time or both feet together, with or without an added bounce. Select the technique that feels best to you.

CALISTHENIC CIRCUIT TRAINING

Calisthenics (from the Greek, meaning beautiful strength) is a series of rhythmic exercises usually performed without apparatus to develop muscular strength, muscular endurance, and flexibility. Because you need little or no equipment, calisthenics allows you to perform your exercises at home or while traveling. As commonly practiced, such exercises are not a well-rounded fitness program. Using the model program based on *circuit training,* however, can increase the value of calisthenics for fitness. This model program consists of twelve exercises.

Terminology

Here are the terms you'll need to know in doing this model program.

Circuit Training   A system of organizing a series of exercises arranged for consecutive performance. Exercises for different muscle groups follow each other, which helps delay the onset of fatigue. When you have performed all twelve exercises in this model program, you have completed one circuit. Three trips around the circuit are required for this model program. Because you're striving for a *target time* (see below), you need to record your time for completing the three trips around the circuit. At first, of course, it takes a longer time to complete the circuit, but as you improve in fitness, you will improve your time (you'll need less rest and your pace will quicken).

Repetitions   The number of times you perform an exercise.

Target Time   For this model program, twenty minutes is the target time—the time within which you hope to complete three circuits. When you hit your target, increase the number of repetitions of each exercise.

Work Description   At first, your work description is one-half of your maximum effort. For example, if you can do 16 push-ups in one minute (your maximum effort), your work description is 8 push-ups in one minute. Performing your exercises at one-half of your maximum effort for three trips around the circuit provides progressive overload. (With a maximum effort of 16 push-ups and a work description of 8 push-ups, you would do 8 push-ups for each of three trips around the circuit for a total of 24 push-ups—8 more than your maximum effort of 16—thus providing progressive overload.) Your work description will increase as you become more fit.

Calisthenic Circuit Training Program

Purpose   To develop and maintain CRE, muscular strength, muscular endurance, and flexibility of the major joints.

Equipment   This model program requires no special equipment. But a stopwatch is useful to record time.

STEP-BY-STEP GUIDE TO CALISTHENICS CIRCUIT TRAINING

1. Learn the twelve exercises described on pp. 135–139. Be able to smoothly perform each exercise in consecutive repetitions.

2. Perform as many arm circles as you can in 30 seconds. Write this number of repetitions in the first max column on the "Calisthenics Circuit Training Record Card." Write half of this number in the work description column labeled "½ max."

3. Perform as many jumping jacks as you can in one minute. Write this number of repetitions in the first max column. Write half of this number in the ½ max column.

4. Repeat instruction 3 for push-ups, then parallel squats, sit-ups, side leg raises, knees-to-chest, alternate toe touches, squat thrusts, shoulder bridges, and side bends. Rest fully between exercises to obtain true maximums.

5. Run in place at the fastest pace you can for three minutes, counting alternate steps (every left or right). Write this number of repetitions in the max column. Write half of this number in the ½ max column.

6. The ½ max column should now be completely filled. You now no longer have to worry about timing the individual exercises.

7. When you are ready to begin calisthenics circuit training, note the time you begin on a clock.

8. Perform the twelve exercises in order, each for the number of repetitions you have written in the ½ max column. (Remember, time no longer matters for each exercise—just work steadily.) Do not rest between the different exercises.

9. When you have completed all twelve exercises at the ½ max number of repetitions (this is one circuit), do two more circuits for a total of three. Do not rest between the circuits.

10. Note the time at the end of the third circuit. Write the date and the total time the three circuits have taken in the columns labeled "time" and "date" on the record card.

11. When you can perform the three circuits in 20 minutes, increase the number of repetitions (the work description) of each exercise by ¼ of the present work description. Write this new number in the next work description column.

12. Use the second set of max and time columns to retest yourself after a period of time has elapsed.

SOURCE: Jerry Goldberg, York College Student Fitness Counselor.

Calisthenics Circuit Training Record Card

Name _____

Exercise	Max	Time	Max	Time	Work Description						
					1/2 Max						
1. Arm circles		30 sec.		30 sec.							
2. Jumping jacks		1 min.		1 min.							
3. Push-ups		1 min.		1 min.							
4. Parallel squat		1 min.		1 min.							
5. Sit-ups		1 min.		1 min.							
6. Side leg raises		1 min.		1 min.							
7. Knee-to-chest		1 min.		1 min.							
8. Alternate toe touch		1 min.		1 min.							
9. Squat thrust		1 min.		1 min.							
10. Shoulder bridge		1 min.		1 min.							
11. Side bend		1 min.		1 min.							
12. Run in place		3 min.		3 min.							

	Time	Date
1		
2		
3		
4		
5		
6		
7		
8		
9		
10		
11		
12		

	Time	Date
13		
14		
15		
16		
17		
18		
19		
20		
21		
22		
23		

Intensity   Determine intensity by testing yourself on each exercise in the circuit to find out how many times you can perform the exercises in the given time. (Testing yourself over a two-day period will reduce the chance of muscle soreness.) You increase intensity by working faster and by increasing repetitions when the twenty-minute target time is achieved. When you can complete three circuits in the target time, increase the repetitions for each exercise by one-fourth of your work description. For example, if your work description is 8 push-ups (one-half of your maximum effort), increase your repetitions to 10 push-ups. Even with this one-fourth increase in repetitions, you should eventually perform the three circuits in the twenty-minute target time. After you have achieved the twenty-minute target time, increase your work description by one-fourth.

Be sure to monitor your pulse rate during the calisthenic circuit so your heart rate stays within your exercise benefit zone. If your heart rate is high, slow your pace.

Duration   Exercise for the length of time it takes you to do three complete circuits. Your aim is to complete three circuits in the target time of twenty minutes, but as you work toward target time, expect to take longer than twenty minutes.

Frequency   Exercise a minimum of three days per week.

At the Beginning

Although a warm-up is intrinsic to the first two exercises in the calisthenic circuit training model program, you should still warm up before you begin each workout (see stretching model program). To establish your work description, test yourself (over two days) to determine how much effort you have to use in order to complete each of the twelve exercises within the time limit. After you have arrived at your work description for each exercise, use it to perform one full circuit for the first three exercise periods. Go on to two full circuits for the next three exercise periods. From then on, each exercise period should consist of three complete circuits. Keep a note pad handy to jot down the date and the time it takes to complete three full circuits. When you can finish three circuits in the target time of twenty minutes, you're ready to increase the repetitions of each exercise and thus increase your work description.

Exercises for Calisthenic Circuit Training Program

Review the instructions on how to perform the exercises in this model program. For best results, do the exercises in the numerical sequence given. Count the number of times you can complete each exercise in the time limit given, and enter that number as your maximum effort. One-half of this is your work description.

When performing the circuit, complete your work description for each exercise as rapidly as possible. When you can do three trips around the circuit in twenty minutes, increase your work description. Doing the circuit as a whole will improve CRE. The body parts affected by the exercises are noted for each part of the circuit, as well as which exercises are especially useful for CRE.

1. **Arm circles: time limit, 30 sec.** (shoulders)
   Holding your arms sideward, palms up, circle forward and then reverse.

   Maximum effort _____

   Work description _____

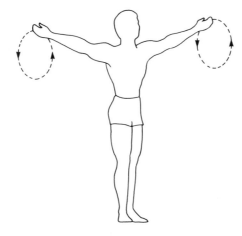

2. **Jumping jack: time limit, 1 min.** (CRE, legs)
   Start with your feet together, jump astride and clap your hands over your head.
   Then jump back to starting position.

   Maximum effort _____

   Work description _____

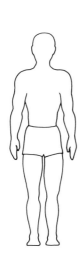
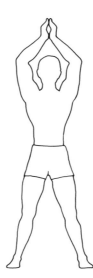

3. **Push-up: time limit, 1 min.** (chest, triceps, upper back)
There are several ways to perform push-ups. The easiest way is to do them against a wall. Stand a straight-arm's distance away from the wall. Keeping your back and legs straight and your heels on the floor, lean forward until your nose touches the wall. Push your body back into a vertical position. Then there is the elevated push-up: First use a table (in place of the wall), then a chair, then an object lower than a chair—say, a box or a footstool. Try these variations, if the traditional floor position is difficult for you. To add resistance, raise your feet and then lower your chest to the floor.

Maximum effort _____

Work description _____

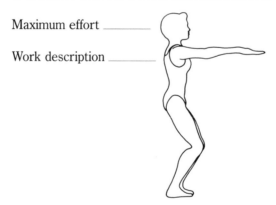

4. **Parallel squat: time limit, 1 min.** (quadriceps, hips)
Keeping your back flat, bend your knees until the top of your thighs are parallel to the floor. Hold for two seconds and return to standing position.

Maximum effort _____

Work description _____

5. **Sit-up: time limit, 1 min.** (abdominals)
There are several ways to perform the sit-up. The easiest way is to use your arms to help push your upper body into the sitting position. Next, you can thrust your arms directly out in front of you while sitting up. Or, if your abdominals are in fairly good shape, you can fold your arms across your chest. The most difficult position for the sit-up is placing your hands behind your head. If you use a slant board and can't do even one sit-up, start with your head at the high end of the board. As the sit-ups become easier, gradually lower the head of the board until

you are doing sit-ups on a level surface. You can increase resistance by doing your sit-ups with your head at the lower end of the slant board. Always perform these exercises with your knees bent.

Maximum effort _____

Work description _____

6. **Side leg raise: time limit, 1 min.** (thighs, hips)
   Raise one leg as high as possible, then return to starting position. Exercise first one side and then the other.

   Maximum effort _____

   Work description _____

7. **Knee-to-chest: time limit, 1 min.** (abdominals, hips, lower back)
   Bend both knees up to your chest. Keep your head down and your arms straight at your sides.

   Maximum effort _____

   Work description _____

8. **Alternate toe touch: time limit, 1 min.** (hamstrings, trunk)
   Bend forward with your knees straight. Touch your right fingertips to your left foot and return to standing position. Bend forward with your knees straight. Touch your left fingertips to your right foot and return to standing position. (Each touch equals 1 repetition.)

   Maximum effort _____

   Work description _____

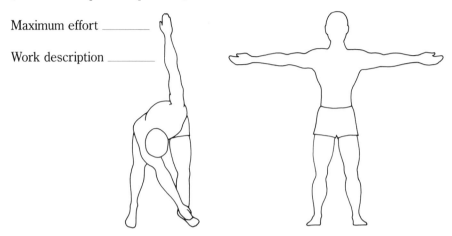

9. **Squat thrust: time limit, 1 min.** (trunk, hips, thighs, arms)
   From a standing position, squat and put your hands on the floor. Thrust both legs backward. Return to the squat position and stand before repeating the exercise.

   Maximum effort _____

   Work description _____

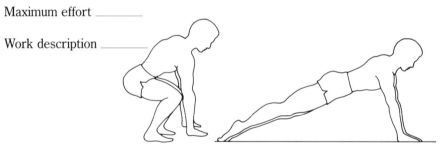

10. **Shoulder bridge: time limit, 1 min.** (lower back)
    Supporting your body on your feet and shoulders, raise your abdomen. Keep both hands behind your head or at your sides and your knees bent.

    Maximum effort _____

    Work description _____

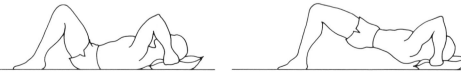

11. **Side bend: time limit, 1 min.** (trunk)
Bend your body to the left (or right). Then reverse. Keep both hands behind your head.

Maximum effort ————

Work description ————

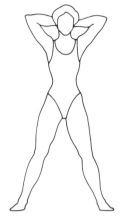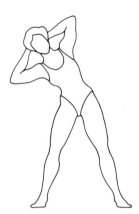

12. **Run in place: time limit, 3 min.** (CRE, legs)

STRETCHING

Stretching develops the flexibility component of physical fitness, and you should include it in the warm-up (before) and cool-down (after) for your fitness program. It can also be a fitness program in itself. We present two stretching model programs here. The first is a basic stretching program of ten exercises that includes movements for most major joints and muscle groups. The second, a ten-part program, is designed as a warm-up/cool-down for most activities, particularly for walking/jogging/running programs, bicycling, and rope skipping.

Terminology

Two terms are important in the stretching model programs.

Static Stretching   To stretch as far as possible without any repetitive bouncing movements. This is the prescribed method of performing each stretching exercise.

Stretch Reflex   A protective contraction of the muscle being stretched. It is the body's defense against overstretch and possible injury.

Basic Stretching Program

Purpose   To develop and maintain flexibility of the major joints of the body.

Intensity and Duration   The intensity and duration for each of the exercises can best be explained in two phases.

1. *The adjustment phase:* Using static stretching, let muscles and other connective tissue gradually get used to the position. By moving slowly and easily into the stretching position, you will avoid the stretch reflex. Allow your body to relax and enjoy the melting away of that tight feeling. Hold the position for ten seconds. As you progress, your body adjusts to the stretching position, and you can gradually increase the time up to thirty seconds. There should be no exertion involved in the adjustment phase.
2. *The development phase:* Repeat the exercise, but now stretch a bit farther. Relax and focus on the pleasurable sensation as your muscles stretch to their limits without pain. Hold the position for fifteen seconds. As you progress, your body becomes accustomed to the stretching position, and you can gradually increase the time up to sixty seconds.

Frequency   To be most effective, do the basic stretching program—which consists of ten exercises involving the major joints and muscle groups—daily.

At the Beginning

Allow your body to move gently and gradually into the stretch position. Stretch slowly and gradually—avoid bouncing. Bouncing sometimes causes injury, usually when momentum builds up and carries the stretch too far. Don't attempt to set records by forcing the stretch to the point of pain.

For the first four or five workouts, allow yourself to become familiar and comfortable with each movement and position. You will get optimal benefit only if you relax and enjoy stretching, whether you use it as a basic stretching program or as warm-up/cool-down.

Exercises for Basic Stretching Program

For best results, do the exercises in the numerical sequence below. We note the body parts affected by the exercises for each part of the stretching program. Stretching is best done after actively warming the muscles.

1. **Shoulder blade scratch** (shoulders, arms)
   Reach back with one arm as if to scratch your shoulder blade. Use your other hand to extend the stretch. Alternate arms.

2. **Towel stretch** (triceps, shoulders, chest)
   Grasp a rolled towel at both ends and slowly bring it back over your head as far down as possible. Keep your arms straight. (The closer your hands are, the greater the stretch.)

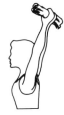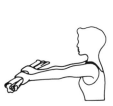

3. **Alternate knee-to-chest** (lower back)
   With hands behind your knees, bring one knee up to your chest. Curl your head toward your knee. Keep the other leg on the floor. Alternate knees.

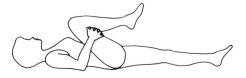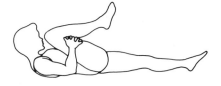

4. **Double knee-to-chest** (lower back)
   Same as alternate knee-to-chest (3), except bring both knees up to your chest.

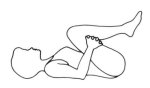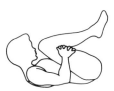

5. **Sole stretch** (groin)
   With the soles of your feet pressed together, pull your feet toward you while pressing your knees down with your elbows.

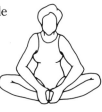

6. **Seated toe touch** (hamstrings)
   Sit with your legs straight. Fold one leg in front and gradually reach for the toes of your other foot. Eventually you will be able to grasp your feet at the instep. Keep your head down. Alternate legs.

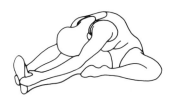

7. **Seated foot-over-knee twist** (hips)
   Seated as depicted, turn at the hips to face the rear. Hold your ankle to keep your foot on the floor. Alternate legs.

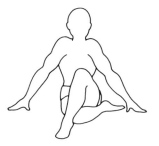 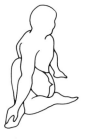

8. **Prone knee flexion** (quadriceps)
   Lying on your side with one arm tucked behind your head, use the other arm to slowly pull one foot up toward your buttocks. Flex the leg up until you feel the stretch in your quadriceps. Alternate legs.

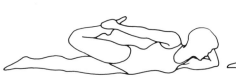 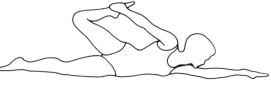

9. **Wall lean** (lower legs)
   Lean against the wall with one leg bent and the other straight. Keep your back straight and your heels on the floor. Bend the knee of the straight leg—this changes the stretch from the calf muscle to the Achilles tendon. Alternate legs.

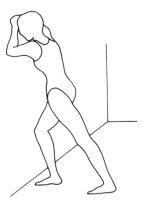 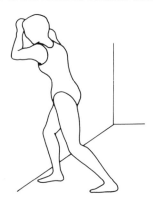

10. **Stride stretch** (hips, hamstring)
    Assume the racer's starting position and stretch one leg backward. Keep your head down. Alternate legs.

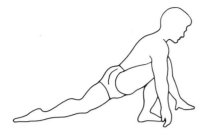
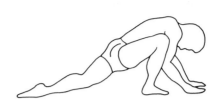

WARM-UP/COOL-DOWN EXERCISES

Do the following exercises before and after most activities—particularly walking/jogging/running programs, bicycling, and rope skipping—to achieve and maintain flexibility. These exercises are done just once, as in the basic stretching program, except for the leg cross-overs and the sit-up, which should be done for 5 to 20 repetitions each. When warming up, precede the following exercises with jumping jacks and three to five minutes of jogging.

For best results, do the exercises in the numerical sequence below. The body parts affected by the exercises are noted for each part of the warm-up/cool-down program.

1. **Alternate knee-to-chest** (abdominals, hips, lower back)
   Bend one knee up to your chest; raise your head and try to touch your knee with your chin. Hold the bent leg with both hands behind your knee. Alternate first one leg and then the other.

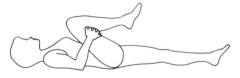
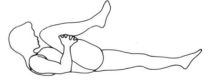

2. **Leg cross-overs** (hips, back)
   Raise one leg and cross it over your body. Keep your upper back flat and your arms extended to the sides. Alternate first one leg and then the other. Turn only your hips.

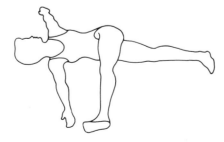

3. **Double knee-to-chest** (lower back)
Same as alternate knee-to-chest (1), except bring both knees up to your chest.

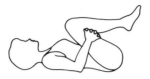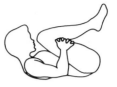

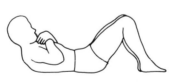

4. **Sole stretch** (groin)
With the soles of your feet pressed together, pull your feet toward you while pressing your knees down with your elbows.

5. **Seated toe touch** (hamstrings)
Sit with your legs straight. Fold one leg in front and gradually reach for the toes of your other leg. Eventually you will be able to grasp your feet at the instep. Keep your head down. Alternate legs.

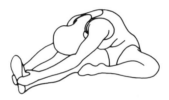

6. **Sit-up** (abdominals)
Cross your arms over your chest as you sit up. Always perform this exercise with your knees bent.

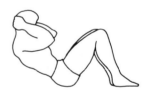

7. **Seated foot-over-knee twist** (hips)
Seated as depicted, turn at the hips to face the rear. Hold your ankle to keep your foot on the floor. Alternate legs.

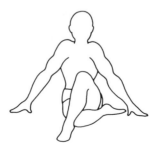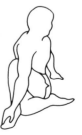

8. **Cat stretch on knees** (upper back, shoulders)
   Resting on your knees, reach forward with one arm and then the other to stretch your shoulders and back.

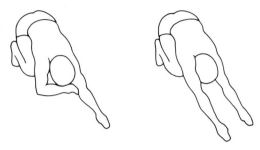

9. **Prone knee flexion** (quadriceps)
   Lying on your side with one arm tucked behind your head, use the other arm to slowly pull one foot up toward your buttocks. Flex the leg up until you feel the stretch in your quadriceps. Alternate legs.

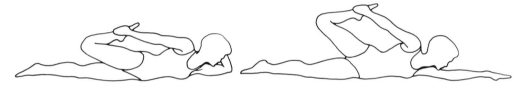

10. **Wall lean** (lower legs)
    Lean against the wall with one leg bent and the other straight. Keep your back straight and your heels on the floor. Bend the knee of the straight leg—this changes the stretch from the calf muscle to the Achilles tendon. Alternate legs.

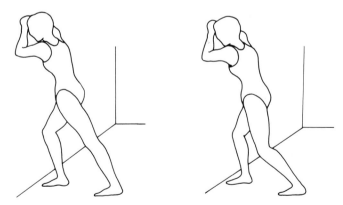

PRINCIPLES OF STRETCHING

- Perform stretching exercises statically. Stretch and hold the position ten to thirty seconds (as long as sixty seconds if your muscles are extremely tight).
- To make stretching exercises more effective, precede them with an isometric contraction of the muscle to be stretched.
- You should feel a mild stretch rather than pain while performing these exercises. Try to relax while stretching.
- Avoid positions that increase the risk of low-back injury. For example, if you are performing straight-leg toe-touching exercises, bend your knees slightly when returning to a standing position.
- As with other forms of physical conditioning, develop flexibility gradually over time.
- There are large individual differences in joint flexibility. Do not feel you have to compete with other athletes during stretching workouts.
- Practice flexibility exercises at least three to five days per week. Set aside a special time to develop this type of fitness.

BICYCLING

Bicycling (or "cycling") can be fun and socially rewarding and can pay large dividends in physical fitness. It is a high–calorie-per-minute activity that promotes changes in body composition and weight control. Fifteen minutes or longer of cycling at a speed fast enough to bring your heart rate into your exercise benefit zone is an excellent exercise for developing a high level of CRE. Also, cycling promotes muscular endurance and muscular strength and improves flexibility of selected muscles of the legs and hips.

For many, cycling is a pleasant and economical alternative to the automobile and a convenient way to improve physical fitness. The advent of 10-speed bikes and their capacity to make uphill pedaling easier has popularized bikes for shopping, going to school and work, and errands. The growing number of bicycle paths and lanes in many communities has also led to more recreational cycling. Cyclists seem to enjoy the freedom provided by the ability to cover long distances easily.

Many cyclists—after a time—join cycling groups on day, weekend, or vacation outings, which can cover hundreds of miles during a tour. (Bicycle racing, however, is a demanding sport that requires a high level of skill and fitness.)

Bicycling Program

Purpose   To develop and maintain all five fitness components by cycling for at least fifteen consecutive minutes with your heart rate within your EBZ.

Equipment   Cycling has its own special array of equipment—including headgear, lighting, safety pennants, and special shoes. But it's the bike itself that requires the largest outlay, ranging from about $100 to as much as $1,000. Avoid a costly investment until you're sure you'll use your bike regularly. Consider renting or borrowing a bike while you investigate what the marketplace has to offer. Don't be influenced by the latest fad or a bike's appearance. The type you buy should be geared to your intended use of the bike. Most cyclists who are interested primarily in fitness are best served by a sturdy 10-speed. A variety of bikes are available, including mountain bikes, which are sturdy with broad tires and up to 21 speeds, and sport and touring bikes, which are less stable, lighter, and faster.

When choosing clothing for bike riding, avoid restrictive or binding garments. But don't wear loose-fitting pants or long skirts that might get caught in the chain. While clothing worn on the upper body should be comfortable and loose, it should not be so loose as to catch the wind and slow you down. You should always use headgear. Some exercisers find a helmet uncomfortable, especially in warm weather. However, preventing a serious head injury makes it worth wearing one. Ideally, the helmet should be equipped with a rear-view mirror.

Intensity, Duration, and Frequency   If you've been inactive for a long time, it may be wise to begin a cycling program at a heart rate that is 10 to 20 percent lower than your EBZ. If your heart rate is too high or if you feel uncomfortable, slow down or stop for a brief rest period (see the following discussion, "At the Beginning"). Once you feel at home on your bike, try a mile at a comfortable speed. Then stop and check your heart rate response by taking your pulse. Don't be concerned if it still falls below your EBZ. After all, it may require several outings to get the muscles and joints of your legs and hips adjusted to this new activity. You should be able to increase your speed gradually, until you can cycle at 12 to 15 miles per hour, a speed fast enough to bring most new cyclists' heart rate into their EBZ. Cycling for at least fifteen minutes three times per week at this speed will lead to improvement in CRE.

When cycling you burn calories, and the more calories you burn the more effective your exercise program. Review Table 7-11 to determine the number of calories that you burn at each outing. You can increase the number of calories burned by cycling faster or for a longer duration. If you can spare the time, it's better to increase distance than to add speed. Don't push too hard. Let your body adapt: Allow your pulse rate to be your guide. More highly fit individuals may need to ride at faster than 13 to 15 miles per hour to achieve heart rates within their EBZ.

Interval training is also effective with cycling. Simply increase your speed for periods of four to eight minutes or for specific distances, one to two miles, say. Then coast for two or three minutes. Repeat the speed interval followed by the slow interval for a total of twenty to sixty minutes, depending on your level of fitness. The slow cycling will allow your heart rate to drop enough to recover in preparation for the next speed interval without a loss in exercise benefits. Cycling over hilly terrain is also a form of interval training: Pedaling uphill is the exercise interval, and coasting downhill is the rest interval.

At the Beginning

Bike riding requires a number of precise skills that practice makes automatic. If you have biked in the past, you will shake off that rusty feeling after a few exploratory

TABLE 7-11   Determining Calorie Cost for Bicycling

This table gives the approximate calorie costs per pound of body weight of cycling from 5 to 60 minutes for distances of .50 mile up to 15 miles on a level terrain. To use the table, find on the horizontal line the time most closely approximating the number of minutes you cycle. Next, locate on the vertical column the approximate distance in miles you cover. The figure at the intersection represents an estimate of the calories used per minute per pound of body weight. Multiply this figure by your own body weight. Then multiply the product of these two figures by the number of minutes you cycle to get the total number of calories burned. For example, assuming you weigh 154 pounds and cycle 3 miles in 20 minutes, you would burn 130 calories: 154 × .042 (calories per pound, from table) = 6.5 × 20 (minutes) = 130 calories burned.

Distance (in miles)	Time (in minutes)											
	5	10	15	20	25	30	35	40	45	50	55	60
.50	.032											
1.00	.062	.032										
1.50		.042	.032									
2.00		.062	.039	.032								
3.00			.062	.042	.036	.032						
4.00				.062	.044	.039	.035	.032				
5.00				.097	.062	.045	.041	.037	.035	.032		
6.00					.088	.062	.047	.042	.039	.036	.034	.032
7.00						.081	.062	.049	.043	.040	.038	.036
8.00							.078	.062	.050	.044	.041	.039
9.00								.076	.062	.051	.045	.042
10.00								.097	.074	.062	.051	.045
11.00									.093	.073	.062	.052
12.00										.088	.072	.062
13.00											.084	.071
14.00												.081
15.00												.097

trips. If you have never ridden, investigate the possibility of a course. (Many courses are not just for the neophyte. They help to develop braking, shifting, and emergency skills and teach ways of caring for and repairing your bike.) Until you become a skilled cyclist, select routes with the fewest hazards and avoid heavy automobile traffic.

Begin each outing with a ten-minute warm-up. (See warm-up/cool-down in stretching model program.) Pay particular attention to stretching the hamstrings because cycling tends to tighten them. Also, do not neglect stretching exercises for the back and neck muscles.

Safety Tips

The National Injury Information Clearinghouse (a federal agency) classifies bicycle riding as the nation's most dangerous sport. Many of the injuries are the result of the cyclist's carelessness. Fred Delong, in his book *Delong's Guide to Bicycles & Bicycling*, suggests that cyclists practice "preventive cycling." The following list is adapted from Delong's recommendations:

- Keep on the correct side of the road. Bicycling against traffic is usually illegal and always dangerous.

- Obey all traffic signs and signals.
- On public roads, ride in single file, except in low-traffic areas (if the law permits). Ride in a straight line; don't swerve or weave in traffic.
- Be alert; anticipate movements of other traffic and pedestrians. Listen for approaching traffic that is out of your line of vision.
- Slow down at street crossings. Check both ways before crossing.
- Use hand signals—the same as for automobile drivers—if you intend to stop or turn. Use audible signals to warn those in your path.
- Maintain full control. Avoid anything that interferes with your vision. Don't jeopardize your ability to steer by carrying anything (including people) on the handlebars.
- Maintain your bicycle in good shape with attachments securely tightened and brakes, gears, saddle, wheels, and tires all in good condition.
- See and be seen. Use a headlight at night; equip your bike with rear reflectors. Use side reflectors on pedals, front and rear. Wear light-colored clothing or use reflective tape at night and bright colors or fluorescent tape by day.
- Be courteous to other road users. Anticipate the worst, and practice preventive cycling.
- Use a rear-view mirror and always wear a helmet.

Common Cycling Ailments

Some cycling ailments are bothersome but easy to prevent. Others should be treated promptly to avoid having to discontinue cycling.

Saddle Soreness   Saddle soreness is due to two conditions: pressure on the soft tissue of the genital area and on the buttocks that may cause pain, tingling, or numbness; and chafing caused by friction on the skin of the buttocks. These problems can be prevented or reduced by the following measures.

Use a comfortable saddle, one that is reasonably soft (or softened with padding or a leather softener). Adjust the saddle to a comfortable height. The height you select should allow your legs to almost reach full extension while pedaling. During long rides, you may find it comfortable to periodically change the tilt of the saddle slightly. Frequently change the position of your body on the saddle. Also adjust the handlebars to change your body position.

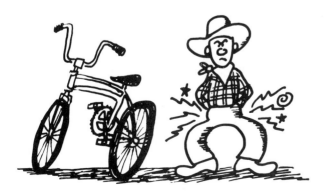

A comfortable saddle can be the key to pleasant cycling.

Wear a pair of cycling pants or shorts padded by soft chamois sewn in the seat to act as a cushion and reduce friction. The liberal use of talcum powder or cornstarch can also reduce friction. It may be wise to carry a supply if you go on a trip. Once irritation has formed, petroleum jelly is useful (though messy). Consult a physician about skin infections.

Numb Hands   Long trips can result in a numbness of the hands. You can try to prevent this by wearing well-padded gloves. You can also pad the handlebars with foam and periodically shift and alter the position of your hands on the handlebars.

Backache and Neck Strain   Beginning cyclists may suffer from backache and neck strain. These may be due to the stretching demands of cycling to which new cyclists are not accustomed. To prevent strains, do exercises designed to stretch the back and neck muscles during your warm-up. In time, the discomfort should disappear.

ROPE SKIPPING

Rope skipping can be an excellent fitness program. It's inexpensive and convenient and an effective exercise for high levels of CRE and muscular endurance of the lower legs. It can also help with weight loss. And it's a fine rainy-day alternative for outdoor CRE activities such as jogging or bicycling.

There are many ways to skip rope, but the most common techniques are jumping on one foot at a time or both feet together, with or without an added bounce. Select the technique that feels best to you. There isn't much difference in the difficulty or energy demands of the various techniques.

At first, you may be grateful to get over the rope in *any* manner. But after a while, skipping rope could become boring if done for long periods of time within the confines of four walls. In time you'll be able to try a variety of approaches—alternating among single jumping on first one foot and then the other, both feet at the same time, crossing your arms over your head, and changing the direction of the rope from front swing to back swing. With a little imagination (and experimentation), you'll be able to create some variations of your own. You could also try skipping rope while watching television or listening to the radio. Some people find that music helps to keep a rhythm.

Rope skipping does little for acquiring and maintaining flexibility. It does develop some strength in the legs and forearms. Because of the muscular demands of rope skipping, it's especially important to warm up adequately. Do stretching exercises for the lower back, lower legs, and hamstrings. (See warm-up/cool-down in stretching model program.)

Terminology

Rope skipping is relatively simple, and so is the language you use.

Turns per Minute   This refers to the number of times the rope passes under your feet in one minute.

Set   One set consists of a combination of an interval of rope skipping for a specific time followed by a rest interval for a specific time.

Rope Skipping Program

Purpose   To develop and maintain CRE and muscular endurance of the lower legs by skipping rope for fifteen minutes (including rest intervals) with your heart rate within your exercise benefit zone.

Equipment   First, there is the rope. Use the correct length (long enough to reach from armpit to armpit, passing under both feet). It can be made of nylon, plastic, hemp, rubber, or leather. Store-bought ropes often come with handles or special grips with weights or ball bearings to use for recording the number of turns. You may find this useful, but start out with clothesline or a simple inexpensive jump rope until you're sure you will continue the exercise. (Jump ropes vary in price from $3 to $15.) Because rope skipping requires constant impact on the metatarsal bones (the ball of the foot), a good pair of jogging shoes may be helpful. In any case, wear comfortable supportive sneakers or running shoes. And a watch or clock is useful to record time.

Intensity and Duration   Rope skipping as a form of interval training uses sets of skipping intervals alternating with rest intervals, gradually increasing the skipping time at the expense of the rest time.

A good starting program for beginning rope skippers is to do one set of fifteen seconds of rope skipping followed by fifteen to thirty seconds of rest. Increase the number of sets gradually as your legs, arms, and CRE begin to make the necessary adjustments. (See Table 7-12 for a sample rope skipping program.) Periodically check your pulse rate so that your heart rate stays within your EBZ: Increase or slow down your turns per minute as needed.

It is important to remember to monitor your heart rate carefully. You may want to keep your heart rate 10 to 20 percent below your EBZ at the beginning. As your condition improves, you will be able to increase your skipping intervals and decrease your rest intervals. Eventually, you may be able to skip rope for fifteen minutes or longer without stopping—even though it is not necessary to do so. You can achieve high levels of CRE and muscular endurance on the interval skipping program. Continue to add skipping/resting sets until your total rope skipping intervals—not counting rest intervals—add up to fifteen minutes. As your CRE and muscular endurance improve, you may find you can increase the intensity (turns of the rope per minute) to keep your heart rate within your EBZ.

Frequency   Because of the constant impact on the feet, it's wise to limit rope skipping to every other day. Or you could alternate it with other forms of CRE exercise such as bicycling, walking, or swimming to limit any trauma to your feet.

At the Beginning

How to skip rope can present a modest challenge to the novice; and even if you've been an active rope skipper in the past, you may find that your legs and arms now tire quickly. Rope skipping is vigorous exercise and too demanding for most sedentary people without a gradual introduction. As with prospective joggers, inexperienced

TABLE 7-12   Sample Rope Skipping Program

This table gives calorie costs for eleven different rope skipping programs. The resting and skipping intervals shown are suggestions only. You can increase or decrease the intervals and the number of sets by one or two as necessary to keep within your EBZ. The approximate calories per pound are for skipping intervals at a rate of 70 turns per minute. (See Appendix B for information about calories burned while rope skipping at 80, 90, and 100 turns per minute.) To find the total calories burned, multiply your weight by the appropriate number of calories per pound. For example, if you skip rope for 3 minutes (first column) with 60-second rest intervals (second column) and you do 6 sets (third column), the total time skipping rope is 18 minutes, and you would burn 1.3 calories per pound. If you weigh 154 pounds, you'd burn approximately 200 calories: 154 × 1.3 (calories per pound, from table) = 200 calories burned.

Skipping interval (minutes: seconds)	Rest interval (minutes: seconds)	Number of sets	Total skipping time (in minutes)	Approximate calories used per pound
0:15	0:30	4–10	1–2.5	.07–.18
0:30	0:30	5–10	2.5–6	.18–.43
0:45	0:30	8–12	6–8	.43–.57
0:60	0:30	6–12	8–12	.57–.86
1:30	0:30	8–10	12–15	.86–1.1
2:00	0:60	8	16	1.2
3:00	0:60	6	18	1.3
6:00	1:30	3	18	1.3
9:00	1:30	2	18	1.3
12:00	2:00	2	24	1.7
15:00	0:00	1	15	1.1

rope skippers should start out with a period of walking to begin the necessary muscular and CRE adjustment to rope skipping. The first step in a rope skipping program for beginners, therefore, should be completing model program 1: walking (starting).

Ease into rope skipping if you have limited skill. Start gradually, allowing muscles and CRE to adjust. Skip on firm but resilient surfaces.

Start by practicing the "rope twirl," by doubling the rope and placing both handles of the rope in one hand. Twirl the rope forward in a circular motion and every time the rope hits the floor, you jump. Practice the rope twirl with the rope in one hand for fifteen seconds, rest fifteen to thirty seconds, then begin the rope twirl again with the rope in the other hand. Once you've mastered the rope twirl, you're ready to start skipping rope. Begin slowly. Select a pace that is comfortable—60 turns per minute should be right for most beginners. As you become more proficient, you will be able to skip from 70 to more than 100 turns per minute.

Many activities designed to promote CRE consist of continued rhythmic activities within your EBZ for at least fifteen minutes. Rope skipping for fifteen uninterrupted minutes, however, presents more muscular stress than other CRE activities (jogging, for example). So it may not even be practical for people with limited muscular endurance or who have muscle and joint problems. What's more, it's difficult to skip rope for fifteen minutes at a rate of 50 to 60 turns per minute and still maintain a rhythm. At that rate, heart rate response for beginners may tend to go beyond the EBZ very quickly. The sample rope skipping program (Table 7-12) is designed to help you keep your heart rate within your EBZ by showing you how to use rest intervals.

SWIMMING

One of the best all-around exercises, swimming is a large-muscle, rhythmic activity that is self-paced. Like jogging and bicycling, it has excellent potential for bringing your heart rate into your exercise benefit zone and thus for developing a high level of CRE.

The most common swimming strokes are the crawl (freestyle), sidestroke, elementary backstroke, breaststroke, and arm-over-arm backstroke. Swimming, using any one or a combination of these strokes for fifteen consecutive minutes, develops muscular strength. Most strokes also encourage shoulder joint flexibility and high levels of muscular endurance. Some people find swimming helpful for changing body composition. It is because swimming develops all five fitness components that it is so highly rated as a well-rounded exercise.

Terminology

The language for this model program is familiar to most swimmers.

Laps   One width or one length of a pool, regardless of pool size.

Swimming Program

Purpose   To develop and maintain all five fitness components by swimming fifteen consecutive minutes with your heart rate within your EBZ.

Equipment   Swimming goggles to protect your eyes from irritation in chlorinated pools.

Intensity and Duration   If you have not been active and have not done any swimming for a long time, begin a swimming program by spending two or three weeks (three times per week) leisurely swimming at a pace that keeps your heart rate 10 to 20 percent below your EBZ. Gradually increase either the duration, the intensity, or both duration and intensity of your swimming to raise your heart rate to a comfortable level within your EBZ, as described below. This can be done by alternating swimming intervals with rest intervals and by gradually increasing the swimming intervals and decreasing the rest intervals.

Calories burned while swimming are the result of the pace: how far you swim and how fast (see Table 7-13).

Frequency   Swim at least three times per week (more often if you want changes in body composition).

SWIMMING EBZ

As a non-weight-bearing, nonupright activity, swimming evokes a lower heart rate per minute during activity. Therefore, intensity should be guided by an adjusted exercise benefit zone. To calculate your EBZ for swimming, simply use this formula:

Maximum swimming heart rate (SHR) = 205 − age
Max. SHR × .70 = lower threshold of EBZ
Max. SHR × .85 = upper threshold of EBZ

TABLE 7-13   Determining Calorie Cost for Swimming

To use this table, find on the horizontal line the distance in yards that most closely approximates the distance you swim. Next, locate on the appropriate vertical column (below the distance in yards) the time it takes you to swim the distance. Then locate in the first column on the left the approximate number of calories burned per minute per pound for the time and distance. To find the total number of calories burned, multiply your weight by the calories per minute per pound. Then multiply the product of these two numbers by the time it takes you to swim the distance (minutes: seconds). For example, assuming you weigh 154 pounds and swim 100 yards in 4 minutes, you would burn 25 calories: 154 × .041 (calories per pound, from table) = . 63 × 4 (minutes) = 25 calories burned.

Calories per minute per pound	Distance in yards					
	25	100	150	250	500	750
.033	1:15	5:00	7:30	12:30	25:00	30:30
.041	1:00	4:00	6:00	10:00	20:00	30:00
.049	0:50	3:20	5:00	8:20	18:40	25:00
.057	0:43	2:52	4:18	7:10	17:20	21:30
.065	0:37.5	2:30	3:45	6:15	10:00	
.073	0:33	2:13	3:20	5:30	8:50	
.081	0:30	2:00	3:00	5:00	8:00	
.090	0:27	1:48	2:42	4:30	7:12	
.097	0:25	1:40	2:30	4:10	6:30	

At the Beginning

Nonswimmers may need a good deal of instruction to develop the necessary skills. (But even the instructional program can be a valuable fitness experience for beginners while teaching them swimming skills.)

A major factor in effective swimming is the ability to breathe rhythmically. With this technique, breathing is coordinated with the stroke—you inhale when your face is out of the water and exhale when your face is submerged. It takes a while for most beginners to learn rhythmic breathing. So if you're serious about your swimming—and if breathing while swimming is a problem for you—it will pay to invest the time and the money for instruction.

If you already know how to swim, and are ready to begin the model program, be sure to start each session with a ten-minute warm-up (see stretching model program).

Start swimming laps of the width of the pool if you can't swim the length. To keep your heart rate below your EBZ, take rest intervals as needed. Swim one lap and rest fifteen to ninety seconds as needed. Start with ten minutes of swim/rest intervals and work up to fifteen minutes. How long it will take you depends on your swimming skills and muscular fitness.

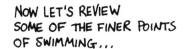

NOW LET'S REVIEW SOME OF THE FINER POINTS OF SWIMMING...

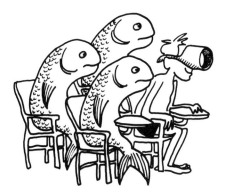

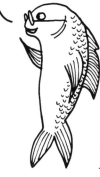

Once you've gotten used to swimming, you'll find it's one of the best all-around exercises.

As You Progress

Once you can swim the length of the pool at a pace that now keeps your heart rate within your EBZ, continue swim/rest intervals for twenty minutes. The rest intervals should be thirty to forty-five seconds. You may find it helpful to get out of the pool during the rest interval and walk for thirty to forty-five seconds, or until you've lowered your heart rate.

Next, swim two laps of the pool length and continue swim/rest intervals for thirty minutes. For the thirty-second rest interval between every two laps, walk (or rest) until you've lowered your heart rate. Gradually increase the number of consecutive swimming laps until you feel ready to try to swim for fifteen minutes without stopping. Select a pace that allows you to keep your heart rate within your EBZ when swimming nonstop for fifteen minutes. At a pace of 20 yards per minute, you will swim about 300 yards; at a 45-yard-per-minute pace, you will cover about 1,000 yards in fifteen minutes. Be cautious about swimming at too fast a pace: It can take your heart rate too high and limit your ability to sustain your swimming.

Varying your strokes can rest your muscles and help prolong the swim. A variety of strokes will also involve more muscle groups and provide a better balanced workout.

Health and Safety Tips

- Swim only in a pool with a qualified lifeguard on duty.
- Dry your ears well after swimming. If you experience the symptoms of swimmer's ear (itching, discharge, or even a partial hearing loss), consult your physician. If you swim while recovering from swimmer's ear, protect your ears with a few drops of lanolin on a wad of lamb's wool.

WEIGHT TRAINING

The most effective means for developing both muscular strength and muscular endurance is weight training—whether you use a weight training machine or free weights, also known as barbells and dumbbells. And this model program of seven exercises will enhance the strength and endurance of all your major muscle groups. The model program requires you to select a weight for each of the seven exercises, performing at least 8 repetitions of each exercise. When you are able to perform 15 repetitions, you increase the weight.

This basic program in progressive weight training is suitable for almost everyone regardless of the level of muscular fitness. You can tailor the program to your level of strength by selecting the amount of resistance you can handle.

People with coronary heart disease, coronary risk factors, or circulatory ailments, however, should consult a physician before beginning a program in weight training. And it must be specially adapted for a person with orthopedic problems (see pp. 84–85).

Terminology

Here are the terms you'll need to know in doing this model program.

Load The total number of pounds lifted during each movement of an exercise, including the weight of the bar, the plates, and the collars (see Equipment).

Resistance A force tending to prevent motion: A ten-pound weight offers more resistance than a five-pound weight. When you increase the resistance (by adding weight to the equipment), your muscles work harder. The harder they work, the stronger they become. This regular increase in resistance provides overload—and this is what results in progress.

Repetitions The number of times you perform an exercise.

Set A series of repetitions for a specific exercise.

Weight Training Program

Purpose To develop and maintain muscular strength and endurance of the major muscle groups.

Equipment   Weight training requires its own unique equipment, usually available at sporting goods stores. (Vinyl-covered weights won't scratch the floor but are bulkier than the cast iron variety and take up more room.)

Bar: A steel bar or pipe 4, 5, or 6 feet long. The middle section of the bar may have a knurled surface to provide friction for gripping.

Barbell: A bar with plates and collars attached.

Collars: Metal rings with set screws used to hold the plates in place on the bar.

Plates: Iron or sand-filled plastic discs with a center hole. These are slipped onto the ends of the bar and secured with collars. Plates are usually available in weights of 1¼, 2½, 5, 10, 20 pounds and up.

Bench: A bench 12 to 16 inches high, 10 to 16 inches wide, and 4 to 6 feet long, preferably padded; used for performing certain exercises.

Intensity and Duration   Start with a load you can handle easily. Always attempt to do as many repetitions as you can—but not less than 8. Perform one set, rest, and perform another set of the same exercise; rest and perform a third set of the same exercise. Then move on to the next exercise. Continue until you have completed all seven exercises. When you can do three sets of 15 repetitions of an exercise, increase the load by adding weight (five pounds for arm exercises and ten pounds for leg exercises). After each increase in load, return to performing three sets of as many repetitions as you can (but not less than 8). Keep on with this system during your workouts until you can perform three sets of 15 repetitions with the new load. Continue this progressive overloading, by increasing weight and repetitions, until you reach the level of strength and endurance you wish. To maintain the strength and endurance you have now achieved, exercise at that level of load and repetitions.

Frequency   Weight training fatigues the muscles so it's wise to rest a day between workouts. If you wish, you may work out every day by exercising the upper body one day and the lower body the next. With this model program, we recommend that you work out every other day.

At the Beginning

Always warm up by doing the "clean-and-press" with a weight light enough so you can easily perform from 10 to 15 repetitions. (Or use the warm-up/cool-down in the stretching model program.) By trial-and-error, establish for each exercise a load light enough to be lifted *with ease* for a set of 8 repetitions. Continue with this load for three to five workouts to allow the joints and muscles to make a gradual adjustment and to avoid soreness and stiffness.

It's a good idea to record the number of repetitions and the load you use at each workout. To do this, adapt Table 7-10, the sample progress chart in the interval circuit training model program.

As You Progress

After you become proficient in weight training, you may want to progress beyond the model program—to work on some specific fitness goal, perhaps. If you want to

TABLE 7-14   Sample Weight Training Progress Card

In this sample, the first column lists the exercises in the model weight training program in the order of performance. Columns for amount of weight and repetitions follow. To assure progressive overload, entries should be made during each workout. This sample is based on a system of 8 to 15 repetitions. Please note that when 15 repetitions are performed, the weight is increased during the next workout.

Date	9/20		9/22		9/24	
Exercise	Wt.	Reps.	Wt.	Reps	Wt.	Reps
1. Warm-up	20	15	20	15	25	12
2. Curl	40	8	40	12	40	12
3. Military press	60	12	60	15	65	10
4. Bent rowing	60	15	65	10	65	11
5. Pullover and press	50	12	50	15	55	9
6. Squat	90	15	95	12	95	13
7. Raise on toes	90	15	95	13	95	13
8. Sit-up	—	20	—	25	—	25

Weight Training Progress Chart

Name _____

Date												
Exercise	Wt.	Reps.	Wt.	Reps.	Wt.	Reps.	Wt.	Reps.	Wt.	Reps.	Wt.	Reps.
1.												
2.												
3.												
4.												
5.												
6.												
7.												
8.												
9.												
10.												

concentrate on *muscular strength,* follow a program of 6 to 8 repetitions. Select a weight with which you can complete a minimum of 6 repetitions; when you can perform 8 repetitions, increase the weight and begin again at 6 repetitions. If you want to concentrate on *muscular endurance,* then follow a program of 15 to 25 repetitions. When you can perform 25 repetitions, increase the weight and begin again at 15 repetitions. To develop both muscular strength *and* muscular endurance, a system of from 8 to 15 repetitions is appropriate. See Table 5-1 in Chapter 5 for a summary of goals and repetitions. This system of progression is based on the concept of "temporary failure." Continue your repetitions until you fail; if you complete the number of repetitions at the upper end of the system, increase the resistance for your next workout. Temporary failure ensures overload.

Weight training can be helpful if you're interested in improving your sports performance. Study the sport to find out which of the muscle groups you should work on. You can then direct your weight training toward the development of the specific muscles involved.

Safety Tips

- Before you begin a workout, be sure the collars and plates on the barbells and dumbbells are tightly secured.
- Use a towel or chalk to keep your hands dry.
- Avoid holding your breath while lifting weights. Get into the habit of inhaling in preparation for the lift and exhaling at the conclusion of the lift.
- Do not lift heavy weights unless you're accompanied by two "spotters," who can help if you lose your balance.
- Be aware of what is going on around you.
- Stay away from people who are doing exercises. Bumping into them could result in injury.
- If you are using a weight machine, make sure the weight pin is securely seated into the weight stack and all pulleys are functional.
- Don't use more weight than you are capable of handling safely.
- Report any equipment malfunctions immediately.
- Always warm up before training.
- Don't exercise if you are ill.

Proper Lifting Techniques   Back pain affects approximately 85 percent of all people at some time during their lives. Often the onset of back trouble can be traced to an incident involving improper lifting techniques. You may possibly avoid back problems by observing the following principles:

- Keep your weight as close to your body as possible. The farther you hold a weight from your body, the more strain there is on your back.
- Do most of your lifting with your legs. The large muscles of the thighs and buttocks are much stronger than those of the back, which are better suited for maintaining an erect posture. Keep your hips and buttocks tucked in.
- When picking up an object from the ground, do not bend at your waist with straight legs because this action places tremendous strain on the lower back muscles and disks.
- Do not twist while lifting. Twisting places an uneven load on back muscles, which can cause strain.

- Lift the weight smoothly, not with a jerking, rapid motion. Rapid motions place more stress on the spinal muscles.
- Allow adequate rest between lifts. Fatigue is a prominent cause of back strain.
- Lift within your capacity. You should not lift a load beyond the limits of your strength.

Spotters   Spotters assist the lifter in the event of a failed repetition, help the lifter move the weight into position to begin a lift, and actively assist with the lift. Use a spotter whenever there is the slightest danger of missing a lift. A weight that gets out of control and falls on you can cause serious injury or death.

Helping a lifter after a failed repetition is a critical responsibility of a spotter. The spotter must quickly recognize that there is a problem and go to the lifter's aid. For inexperienced weight trainers, it is best to have two spotters for most lifts. More experienced lifters prefer only one spotter because they are more predictable.

Spotters must be careful not to injure themselves. Spotters should observe proper lifting techniques: bend the knees, maintain a straight back, and keep the weight close to the body. The lifter should not give up on the lift completely and should assist the spotter in putting the bar back on the rack.

Spotters should be attentive, but not so much that they disrupt the lifter's concentration. When spotting, try to stay out of the lifter's field of vision as much as possible, but follow the path of the bar closely enough so that you can step in if the lifter can't complete the exercise.

Weight Training Exercises

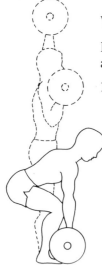

For best results, do the exercises in the numerical sequence given. The body parts affected by the exercises are noted for each.

1. **Warm-up: clean-and-press** (full body)
   Lift the barbell from the floor to your chest in one movement and then push it over your head, using only your arms.
   Safety: Be sure your knees are bent and your back is flat when lifting the barbell from the floor.

2. **Curl** (biceps, forearms)
   With your palms forward and elbows close to your sides, bend your elbows, bringing the barbell up to your chest. Do not swing your body forward and back. Maintain a stationary position. When performing this exercise on a Universal gym, stand as close to the machine as possible. Adjust the chain so that you have resistance throughout the range of motion.

Caution: Using a straight bar can cause strain of the forearm muscles in some people. If you have a problem, consider using a "curl bar" for this exercise because it places less stress on the forearms.

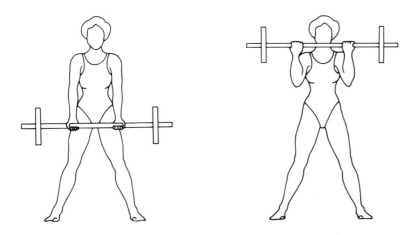

3. **Military press** (upper back, shoulders, arms)

   From your shoulders push the barbell over your head, using only your arms. When you are performing this lift on a Universal or Nautilus machine, make sure you are sitting close enough to the machine so that you are pushing up rather than out.

   Safety: Push the barbell directly or slightly backward over your head so that it is in line with your center of gravity. Do not arch your back excessively, or you may injure the spinal muscles, vertebrae (bones of the spine), or disks.

   Spotters: This lift requires two spotters. Spotters should stand on both sides of the weight.

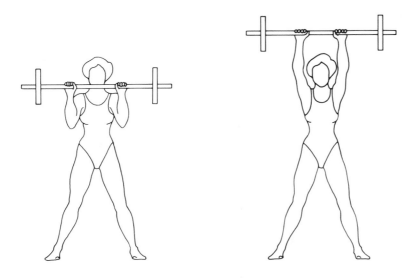

4. **Bent rowing** (upper back, arms)

With your back flat and knees bent, raise the barbell to your chest, keeping your elbows high.

Safety: Do this exercise while resting your head on a table to protect your back.

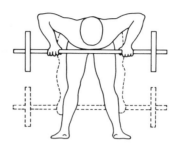

5. **Bent arm pullover and press** (upper back, chest, triceps)

Grasp the bar with your palms forward and your hands as wide apart as possible. Keeping your elbows bent, pull the bar directly to a resting position on your chest. Push the bar straight up from your chest. Lower the barbell to your chest and then return it slowly to the floor.

Safety: Control the weight so it doesn't strike your face.

Spotters: Stand directly behind lifter. Be particularly watchful of the weight hitting the lifter's throat.

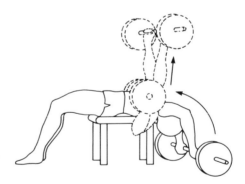

6. **Parallel squat** (quadriceps, hips)

With the barbell resting on the back of your shoulders, lower your body by bending at the knees. In the squat position, the top of your thighs should be parallel with the floor.

Safety: Keep your back flat and head up. Never bounce at the bottom of the squat because this might cause injuries to the ligaments of your knees.

Spotters: This lift requires two spotters. Spotters should stand on both sides of the weight.

The leg press, a variation of this exercise, can be done on a Universal gym. Adjust the seat so that your knees are bent to at least a 45-degree angle. Make sure your back is flat against the back of the chair. Extend your legs to perform this exercise.

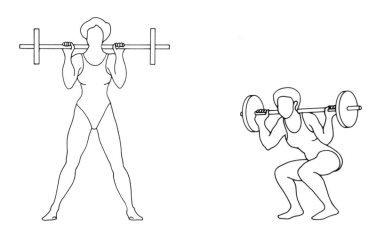

7. **Raise on toes** (lower legs)
   With the barbell resting on the back of your shoulders, stand with the balls of your feet on a two-inch board. Raise your heels from the floor and return.
   Spotters: A spotter should stand at both sides of the bar, slightly to the rear of the lifter.

   Toe presses, a variation of this exercise, can be done on a Universal gym. After performing leg presses, extend your knees fully so that your legs are straight. Press down with your toes.

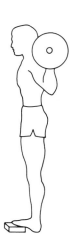 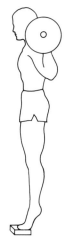

8. **Sit-up** (abdominals)

Cross your arms on your chest as you perform the sit-up. You can increase resistance by doing your sit-ups with your head at the lower end of a slant board. Always perform these exercises with your knees bent.

Caution: If you have neck problems, do not do this exercise with your hands behind your head because you may put too much pressure on the disks in the upper spine and on fragile neck muscles.

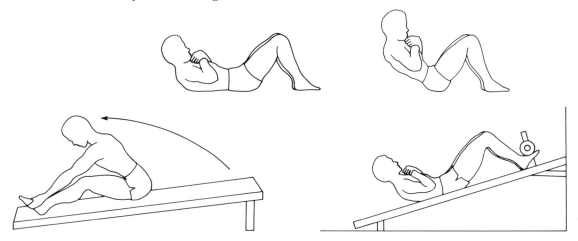

EQUIPMENT FOR A HOME EXERCISE CIRCUIT

For many exercisers, the fully equipped commercial gymnasium or the lure of the outdoors is exciting and stimulating. Fortunately, there's an alternative if you prefer privacy during your attempts to improve physical fitness: You can set aside space at home for exercising. In fact, most home exercisers don't need very much space. And some exercise programs don't even need any store-bought equipment at all. With ordinary items found in any home, you can develop a circuit training program (based on the interval circuit training model program) that can benefit all the components of physical fitness.

Some households already have exercise equipment available. The stationary bicycle, for example, can form the basis for a useful circuit training program.

No equipment or program can provide fitness benefits, however, unless used correctly on a regular basis. To do this, a person must observe the principles of progressive overload (intensity, duration, and frequency) and specificity. To develop and maintain physical fitness, a program using household items or equipment must meet certain criteria.

• *Cardiorespiratory endurance (CRE):* Equipment is useful for CRE if it offers the opportunity to exercise within your EBZ for a minimum of fifteen minutes. Usually the exercise must involve the body's largest muscle groups—the legs (including thighs) and the back.

- *Body composition:* Equipment for improving body composition must allow you to burn a high number of calories during one exercise session, which should last thirty minutes or more.
- *Muscular strength:* To develop muscular strength, the equipment must be capable of supplying sufficient resistance for 6 to 8 repetitions during maximum effort.
- *Muscular endurance:* Muscular endurance equipment must allow you to perform at least 15 repetitions, with the potential of increasing to 25 repetitions or more during maximum effort.
- *Flexibility:* To be considered useful, equipment for improving flexibility must permit movement through the full range of motion of the joints.

If you already have it on hand, you might like to use in a circuit training program the store-bought exercise equipment described below.

Stationary Exercise Bicycle

In January 1982 *Consumer Reports* reported on a total of eighteen models of single-action stationary bicycles. Exercise on a single-action bike is pedaling, as on a regular bike. The stationary bike is capable of promoting CRE and muscular endurance of the leg muscles. By providing variable pedaling resistance to the needs of the exerciser, it can require sufficient effort of the large muscle groups of the legs to push the heart rate into the exercise benefit zone (EBZ). Because pedaling can burn a lot of calories, regular use should also contribute to the loss of body fat. Check your pulse rate regularly when you start the program to find out if you're pedaling hard enough to stay within your EBZ.

Another type of stationary exercise bike is the motorized model that generates a coordinated movement of the pedals, seat, and handlebars. It may operate at one or two rates of speed. The most productive way of using this model is to attempt to push, pull, and pedal as if to speed up the action—even though you really can't make it go faster.

If used regularly, the motorized stationary bike can develop CRE as well as many muscle groups. The most effective approach is use of an interval training system. For example, you may pull, push, and pedal for ten to fifteen seconds and then let the motor take over for fifteen to thirty seconds of relief interval. At first you may let the bike do much of the work. In time, however, you should find that the intensity and duration of active push, pull, and pedal intervals will increase.

Rowing Machine

The rowing machine is designed to simulate the action of competitive rowing. Handles are available as "oars," usually with increments to decrease or increase resistance. The feet are generally strapped to foot rests to ensure strong leg action (particularly of the quadriceps but also of the hamstrings).

You can maintain your heart rate within your EBZ if you extend your legs vigorously and your arms and back are fully active. Vary the pace to ensure adequate intensity and duration. In addition to its CRE value, the rowing machine can develop muscular endurance in the arms, upper and lower back, and legs. Rowing can also promote flexibility of most of the joints.

Allow time for your muscles to become conditioned to the movement of rowing. Begin with a few minutes of slow-paced rowing without concern for reaching your EBZ. At a comfortable rowing pace, gradually increase duration over a period of several weeks. Then try to reach your EBZ and to prolong your duration for a minimum of fifteen minutes.

If you have high blood pressure or orthopedic or circulatory problems, you should get medical clearance before beginning an exercise program based on the rowing machine.

Treadmill

As a result of significantly lower prices, motorized treadmills designed for home use are now readily available. These treadmills allow you to adjust both speed and angle of incline. This means that you can walk or jog on level ground or uphill.

You should begin your exercise program at a very low intensity and gradually increase your workload during a single exercise session as well as over a period of weeks and months. Warming up, followed by weight training exercises or calisthenics, and finishing up your workout on the treadmill can provide you with a well-rounded exercise program.

Like the stationary bicycle and the rowing machine, the motorized treadmill is a good choice for yearround CRE exercise, regardless of the weather.

Nordic Skiing

Cross-country skiing is one of the finest CRE exercises you can select. The good news is that you don't need snow to enjoy the benefits of this activity.

You can ski outdoors on dry land using roller skis. These devices are simply short skis with a front and back wheel; ski poles are used, and the motion and muscle groups are exactly as they would be when skiing on snow. Another position is to ski indoors on a cross-country ski machine, which allows you to simulate the activity with all of its CRE and muscular benefits.

As cross-country can be a very strenuous activity, it is advisable to start at a slow or moderate pace with limited duration and gradually increase over a period of time.

Jump Rope

The jump rope, whether fancy handled or just a piece of clothesline, is a useful device for developing CRE and muscular endurance of the lower legs. Because rope skipping is relatively high in calorie cost, it can improve body composition. (See rope skipping model program.)

Stair Climber

It is well known that climbing stairs can get you huffing and puffing, which is the hallmark of a good CRE activity. The large muscle groups of the hips and thighs carry the workload and thus receive much of the benefits.

Stepping up and down on a bench or box (as described on p. 130) is an excellent CRE exercise requiring nothing more than an 18- to 20-inch-high box. Stepping at 20 cycles per minute will burn as many calories as if you had walked 3.5 miles in 56 minutes.

There are also a number of stair-climbing machines that are compact and priced right for home use. Some of these machines allow tension and speed adjustment. Most are equipped with a timer.

Stair climbing, whether on real stairs, a bench, or a machine, can be extremely vigorous depending on your pace. The faster the pace, the more calories will be burned.

Begin stair climbing at low intensity and short duration, and gradually build up over a period of time. As with other CRE programs, be sure to warm up and cool down properly.

Cables

Originally known as "chest expanders" and sometimes called "spring exercisers," this inexpensive piece of equipment may consist of as few as three and as many as ten strands of steel springs attached to handles. The device often comes with five springs that you can remove or add in order to adjust the resistance. Cables can develop muscular strength and muscular endurance of the arms, chest, shoulders, and upper back. You can also improve flexibility of the chest and shoulder muscles.

Slant Board

Frequently called an abdominal board, the slant board increases resistance while doing sit-ups with the foot end of the board raised: The higher the angle, the greater the difficulty of the sit-up. The board can also be used for leg, hip, and back exercises. (By raising both ends of the board off the floor—by placing it on chairs, for instance—the slant board can serve as an exercise bench for weight training exercises.)

Wrist Roller

This is an excellent device for developing muscular strength and muscular endurance of the wrists and forearms. Attach a rope to a two-inch dowel (or broomstick). Tie a weight—a size you can handle easily—to the end of the rope. Hold the dowel with one hand at each end (with the rope and weight in the center of the dowel). With your arms either horizontally straight in front of you or bent at the elbow, lower the weight by unwinding the rope, rotating the dowel away from the body. Then bring the weight back up by rewinding the rope around the dowel. Reverse the procedure to vary the exercise.

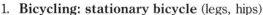

CIRCUIT TRAINING USING AVAILABLE HOME EXERCISE EQUIPMENT

Although the circuit below focuses on a stationary bicycle, it could just as easily focus on a rowing machine, a nonmotorized treadmill, or a jump rope. This circuit can last for durations ranging from fifteen minutes to one hour by adjusting the number of trips around the circuit and by increasing the time on the stationary bicycle. Follow the interval circuit training model program—thirty seconds of exercise followed by fifteen seconds of rest. If you want to emphasize CRE, increase each set of cycling: Instead of thirty seconds, do two to five minutes. (Use miles instead of repetitions for cycling.) CRE is improved by cycling and by the circuit as a whole.

1. **Bicycling: stationary bicycle** (legs, hips)

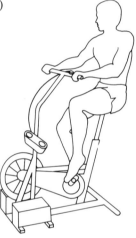

2. **Overhead pull: cables** (upper back, chest)
   With your arms up and diagonally outward, pull your arms horizontally downward to the side until the cables touch the front of your chest. Palms can be inward or outward.

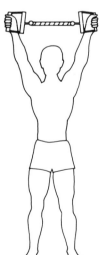

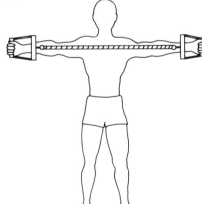

3. **Sit-up: slant board** (abdominals)
   Increase resistance by doing your sit-ups with your head at the lower end of the slant board. Always perform these exercises with your knees bent.

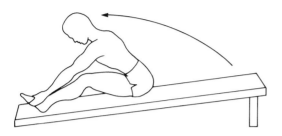
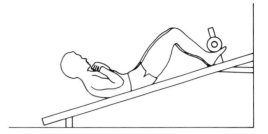

4. **Bicycling: stationary bicycle** (legs, hips)

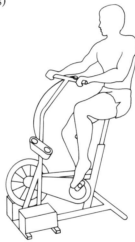

5. **Archer's exercise: cables** (upper back, triceps)
   With your arms straight out in front of you, stretch first one arm then the other horizontally to the side; alternate these movements.

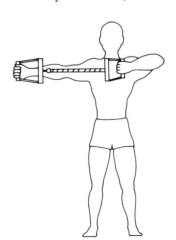
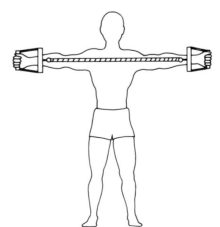

6. **Back extension** (lower back)
Raise your head and shoulders. Keep your legs straight and your hands behind your head.

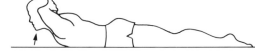

7. **Bicycling: stationary bicycle** (legs, hips)

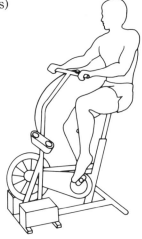

8. **Push-up** (chest, triceps, upper back)
To add resistance, raise your feet and then lower your chest to the floor.

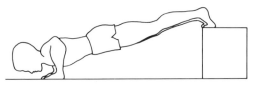

9. **Wrist flexion: wrist roller** (wrists, forearms)
Hold the dowel with one hand at each end (with the rope and weight in the center of the dowel). With your arms either horizontally straight in front of you or bent at the elbow, lower the weight by unwinding the rope, rotating the dowel away from the body. Then bring the weight back up by rewinding the rope around the dowel. Reverse the procedure to vary the exercise.

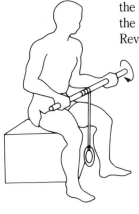

OTHER HOME EXERCISE EQUIPMENT

Not all home exercise equipment can become the focus for a circuit training program. But you can use the kinds of home exercise equipment described below to help you improve fitness.

Chest Crusher

Very useful for developing the muscles of the chest (pectorals), the chest crusher also involves the biceps and shoulders to some extent. Sometimes erroneously called "a bust developer," it actually affects the muscles that serve as a foundation to and support for the breasts.

Chinning Bar

This is a useful and inexpensive piece of equipment. Some store-bought types can be attached to the wall and others can be placed in a doorway (they telescope to require no screws or bolts). Another alternative is to mount a homemade bar in the rafters of your attic or in the basement.

Chinning exercises can enhance muscular strength and muscular endurance of the arms, chest, upper back, and trunk. Relaxed hanging by the hands (with some slow twisting and stretching) can improve flexibility of the shoulders and upper back. For a balanced program, CRE activities would also be necessary.

Doorknob Exerciser

This is a device that attaches to a doorknob with a pulley so that the exerciser can pull with one handle of the rope while resisting with the other. The value in terms of muscular strength and muscular endurance depends on the exercise. Simply going through motions is a waste of time, but actively pulling and resisting can influence muscular endurance and to some extent muscular strength. The device has little or no value for any other fitness component.

Exercise Wheel

The exercise wheel is a device that is marketed to "trim your tummy." If used properly, it can improve muscular strength and muscular endurance of your abdominal muscles, chest, and upper back. It will not result in spot reduction of body fat—there's no such thing. But it will improve the firmness of your abdominal muscles.

The exercise wheel consists of a dowel used as an axle inserted through the center of a solid wheel (sometimes two wheels). Kneel on the floor so that the axle is in line with your shoulders and grasp the axle. Raising your head, inhale and extend your arms forward, rolling the wheel out as far as you can reach comfortably. Exhale slowly and hold the outstretched position for a second or two. Then inhale slowly as you roll the wheel back to starting position.

When first using this piece of equipment, limit the extent of the movement. (You could fall on your face.) It's also wise for a beginner to do only 3 to 5 repetitions to avoid muscle soreness. The exercise wheel forces the abdominal muscles to function as stabilizers of the trunk in a way that does not occur in most calisthenics. By limiting the extent of the movement, you can prevent injury to the lower back.

Grip Exerciser

This piece of equipment can develop the muscular strength and muscular endurance of your grip—depending on the tension of the particular model. If your sports interest requires strong wrists and forearms, as in tennis or handball, this device may be helpful.

Some people keep a grip exerciser in their car and use it when caught in traffic or at stop lights. (It can be an effective way to release tension.) Others use it while watching television or riding a stationary bicycle.

8

Model Weight Loss Program

After you've read this chapter, you will be able to:

List your reasons for wanting to slim down.

Determine how much weight you need to lose.

Assess your daily calorie balance.

Develop a personal contract to guide program activity.

Plan well-balanced menus that are consistent with your daily calorie intake goals.

Plan an exercise program to achieve your calorie output goals.

Record program progress.

Identify steps to maximize program compliance.

As we saw in Chapter 4, efforts to alter your body composition or to control your weight are best achieved by a combination of diet and exercise. As is the case with starting and maintaining an exercise program, altering your eating behavior may not be a simple matter. Your food choices are usually based on a complex relationship of habit and personal preference developed over many years.

Crash diets generally fail because they are nutritionally flawed and do not permanently alter your lifelong approach to eating or exercise. The evidence is clear that more lasting weight control results are achieved by incorporating new eating and physical activity patterns into everyday living. Successful programs include exercise along with a diet composed of a variety of foods from the "daily food guide" (Table 6-5)—but with reduced portion sizes.

The model weight loss program in this chapter uses a "Food Exchange Plan" (see Appendix C) consistent with the "daily food guide" but offering a clear-cut system for planning interesting meals with enough variety for most people's tastes. This model program simplifies menu design to ensure compliance with your personal calorie requirements. Follow the seven steps and use the worksheets to develop your personalized weight loss program.

STEP 1   Reasons for wanting to lose weight.
STEP 2   Choosing weight loss and negative-calorie-balance goals.
STEP 3   Assessing your current calorie balance.
STEP 4   Developing a personal contract.
STEP 5   Planning your weekly menus.
STEP 6   Keeping a record of your progress.
STEP 7   Tips for managing common eating problems.

STEP 1: REASONS FOR WANTING TO LOSE WEIGHT

Ask yourself: Why do I really want to slim down? Establish your personal reasons for wanting to commit yourself to a program that will help you on the road to permanent slimness. Your reasons must be vitally important to you—or you are likely to fail. In

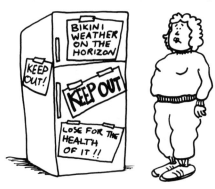

Remind yourself of the reasons you want to lose weight.

TABLE 8-1   Reasons to Lose Weight

Importance	Priority
_____ Follow my doctor's advice	_____
_____ Wear a smaller clothing size	_____
_____ Improve my appearance	_____
_____ Feel more assured and attractive	_____
_____ Feel healthier and more in control of myself	_____
_____ Firm up muscle tone	_____
_____ Improve sports performance	_____
_____ Please someone who is important to me	_____
_____ Help reduce low back pain	_____
_____ Lower high blood pressure	_____
_____ Lower cholesterol and/or triglyceride levels	_____
_____ Increase high-density lipoprotein cholesterol	_____
_____ Help control diabetes	_____
_____ Save more energy and increase stamina	_____
_____ Reduce risk of circulatory disease	_____

Table 8-1, identify the reasons that are important by placing a check in the left column. Assign priorities to those you check by placing a number in the right column. Number 1 is most important, 2 is next, and so on.

You should post the two or three most important reasons where they will be in full view. Suggestions include your car dashboard, your bathroom mirror, and your refrigerator door.

STEP 2: CHOOSING TENTATIVE WEIGHT-LOSS AND NEGATIVE-CALORIE-BALANCE GOALS

Efforts at altering body composition require an increase in the ratio of muscle to body fat. You will almost always need to reduce your weight if you are overfat. By identifying an ultimate target weight and the number of pounds that you need to lose and then determining the negative-calorie-balance program you must adhere to, you will be taking important steps toward altering your body composition.

Ideally, your ultimate target weight should be based on a body fat assessment. Use Profile 8-1A to calculate your ultimate target-weight and negative-calorie goals.

If you have not calculated your percent body fat, Profile 8-1B provides an alternate method for determining your ultimate target-weight and negative-calorie-balance goals.

Once you are clear about your weight-loss and negative-calorie-balance goals, it will be necessary for you to determine exactly why you have accumulated more body fat than you would like to carry. Obviously you have developed a positive calorie balance that has resulted in the storage of excess fat. Either your calorie intake is too great or your calorie output is too little. Most likely the culprit is a combination of the two.

STEP 3: ASSESSING YOUR CURRENT CALORIE BALANCE

To obtain reasonable estimates of your usual calorie balance (the relationship of your calorie intake to output), log all the foods that you eat as well as your physical activity for one week. Profile 8-2, your "Calorie Intake Log," allows you to record all the food you eat each day. It can also help to make you more aware of your diet's nutritional balance as well as the various patterns connected to your eating behavior. Duplicate as many of these worksheets as you need.

Profile 8-3, your "Calorie Output Log," allows you to estimate the total number of calories you burn each day. Duplicate as many as you need so you can maintain records for one week of activity.

To calculate your weekly calorie balance, note your intake and output figures in Profile 8-4, "Weekly Calorie Balance Form."

STEP 4: DEVELOPING A PERSONAL CONTRACT

A written contract can help to clarify what you are going to do to achieve your goals, and it will also enable you to make a more complete commitment, one that you are more likely to carry out. To develop your contract, follow the instructions for completing Profile 8-5, "A Personal Weight Control Contract."

STEP 5: PLANNING YOUR WEEKLY MENUS

By planning your weekly menus, you are more likely to stick to your daily calorie goals. However, calories are not your only concern; it is essential that your menus be nutritionally balanced. To complete Profile 8-6, "Plan Your Weekly Menus," you will also be using Table 8-2 ("Portions Allowed from Each Food Group by Calorie Plan"), Table 8-3 ("Calories per Portion"), and Appendix C ("Food Exchange Plan").

EXAMPLES OF SELF-TALK

Negative

Oops! I ate that piece of cake—that blows today. I'll start again tomorrow.

I always blow it on weekends, at parties, and after dinner.

I don't have time to keep records. I can remember everything anyway.

I goofed again. I can't do it. I might as well give up.

Positive

I'll start back on track right now. A small mistake isn't going to throw me off my program.

I can choose what happens to me by taking responsibility for planning ahead.

Weight management is my first priority, so I'll keep the records.

I can learn from this mistake. I know how to pick up the pieces.

Whenever you sense negative self-talk, shout "No!!!" and turn quickly to positive thoughts.

TABLE 8-2   Portions Allowed from Each Food Group by Calorie Plan

Calorie Plan	Meat	Fat	Bread	Milk	Vegetable	Fruit	Miscellaneous
1,000	3	3	3	2	4	3	—
1,200	6	3	4	2	5	3	1
1,500	7	4	5	3	5	4	2
1,800	7	5	7	3	6	5	2
2,100	9	6	8	4	7	5	2

TABLE 8-3   Calories per Portion

Food group	Portion size	Calories
Meat exchange		
Lean meat	1 ounce	55
Medium-fat meat	1 ounce	78 (omit ½ fat exchange)
High-fat meat	1 ounce	100 (omit 1 fat exchange)
Fat exchange	*	45
Bread exchange	*	70
Milk exchange	*	80
Vegetable exchange		
Group A	½ cup	25
Group B	*	25
Fruit exchange	*	40
Miscellaneous exchange	*	50 (try to avoid; no nutritional value)
Free foods	*	0
Bonus foods	*	110–210 (limit to two times per week)

*See Appendix C, "Food Exchange Plan," for size of portion.

YOUR FITNESS PROFILE 8-1A
Identifying Weight-Loss and Negative-Calorie-Balance Goals
(When Percentage of Body Fat Is Known)

Objective: To set weight-loss and negative-calorie-balance goals.

Directions: Review pp. 18 and 19 in Chapter 1 to determine your current level of body fat and the extent to which you need to alter that percentage. Use the formulas below to calculate your ultimate target-weight and negative-calorie goals.

1. _____ = _____ − _____
   % body fat to be lost   % current body fat   Target % body fat

2. _____ = _____ × _____
   Pounds to lose   % body fat to be lost   Current weight

3. _____ = _____ − _____
   Target body weight   Current weight   Pounds to lose

4. _____ = _____ ÷ _____
   Number of weeks to   Total pounds to lose   Pounds to lose each week
   achieve target weight

5. _____ = _____ × 3,500
   Negative-calorie balance to   Pounds to lose each week
   achieve each week

YOUR FITNESS PROFILE 8-1B
Identifying Weight-Loss and Negative-Calorie-Balance Goals
(Using Height-Weight Tables)

Objective: To set weight-loss and negative-calorie-balance goals.

Directions: Determine your body build using Profile 1-4 in Chapter 1. Then, using the height-weight tables in Appendix A, fill in the following formulas.

1. _____ = _____ − _____

    Pounds to lose   Current weight   Target weight (charts,
                                                                                           p. 256)

2. _____ = _____ ÷ _____

    Number of weeks to   Total pounds to lose   Pounds to lose each week
    achieve target weight

3. _____ = _____ × 3,500

    Negative-calorie balance to   Pounds to lose each week
    achieve each week

YOUR FITNESS PROFILE 8-2
Calorie Intake Log

Objective: To make you aware of when, what, and how much you eat.

Directions:

1. Record the time of day that you eat the food in column 1.

2. Describe the food in column 2. Don't forget the details—the butter on the bread, the sugar in the coffee, and so on.

3. Note the amount of food you eat in column 3. This is usually noted by the general size or weight of the serving. See Appendix C for the serving designations and calorie equivalents of a large variety of foods.

4. Write the number of calories contained in a specific food serving in column 4. Appendix C lists the calorie costs of most foods by their exchange categories.

5. Include comments related to your mood or hunger level and other circumstances connected to food intake in column 5. For example, you might use words or comments such as "anxious," "very hungry," or "snack."

6. Calculate the total number of calories that you take in, and at the end of each day note the total on Profile 8-4, "Weekly Calorie Balance Form."

Daily Intake Log

1 Time	2 Food	3 Amount	4 Calories	5 Comments

Total calorie intake: _____.

PROFILE 8-2

YOUR FITNESS PROFILE 8-3
Calorie Output Log

Objective: To make you aware of how active or sedentary you are.

Directions:

1. Under the activity column, list all your physical activities for the day. For purposes of this worksheet, physical activity refers to all sport and fitness activities as well as other active movement that generates at least .02 calorie per pound per minute. You can find a partial listing of common nonsport activities that fit into this category in Profile 4-2 (in Chapter 4). It is not necessary to list your sedentary activities such as sleeping and eating; they burn less than .02 calorie per minute per pound and are lumped together in the sedentary activity category.

2. Place under column 2 the calorie cost per minute per pound for each of the physical activities you listed in the activity column. You will find the appropriate calorie costs for most of these activities in Profile 4-1 and Profile 4-2 in Chapter 4 and in Appendix B.

3. All your sedentary activities have been lumped together and assigned an average value of .01 calorie per minute per pound.

4. Place the total number of minutes of activity under column 3 alongside each of the physical activities listed.

5. Calculate the total number of minutes to place under column 3 alongside the sedentary category by adding up all the minutes of physical activity and subtracting the amount from 1,440 (the total number of minutes in a day).

6. Note your body weight under column 4 alongside each of the physical activities and the sedentary category.

7. To determine your total calorie output for each of the physical activities as well as for the sedentary activity, under column 5, you must multiply column 2 by column 3 by column 4.

8. To obtain your calorie output for the entire day, total all the figures under column 5.

9. You should note the total number of calories you burn each day on Profile 8-4, "Weekly Calorie Balance Form." If your logs of calorie intake and output are typical of your weekly pattern, a review of Profile 8-4 will enable you to assess whether you have a negative or positive calorie balance. It can also guide you in determining how to adjust that balance to reach a new negative balance.

Daily Output Log

1 Activity	2 Cal./min./lb.	×	3 Total minutes	×	4 Body weight	=	5 Output
1.		×		×		=	
2.		×		×		=	
3.		×		×		=	
4.		×		×		=	
5.							
6.							
7.							
8.							
Sedentary	.01	×		×		=	

Total calorie output: _____ .

YOUR FITNESS PROFILE 8-4
Weekly Calorie Balance Form

Objective: To make you aware of how many calories you use in the course of a week.

Directions: Insert in this profile the intake and output figures you gathered in Profiles 8-2 and 8-3.

Weekly Balance

	Sun.	Mon.	Tues.	Wed.	Thurs.	Fri.	Sat.
Calories in							
Calories out							
Daily difference							
Weekly difference							

STEP 6: KEEPING A RECORD OF YOUR PROGRESS

There are a number of simple methods available to maintain records of your progress. If you keep it regularly, Profile 8-4, "Weekly Calorie Balance Form," can reinforce your efforts. In addition, Profile 8-7, "Weight Control Progress Graph," is a simple method of charting your weight.

STEP 7: TIPS FOR MANAGING COMMON EATING PROBLEMS

Eat Regular Meals and Planned Snacks

A major cause of overeating is irregular eating, marked by skipped meals and then overeating at other times. Another destructive pattern is constant snacking at the expense of regular meals. By using your menu planner, you are more likely to limit yourself to three regularly planned meals and to include the kind of snacks that do not undermine your efforts to alter your body composition.

Choose the Right Foods

The nemesis of many individuals with weight problems is constantly eating one or more high-calorie foods. Usually sweets in the form of candies, ice cream, sugar-laden soft drinks, or taste treats such as potato chips and peanuts are the culprits. If you must snack, develop a taste for and have available a supply of nutritious, low-calorie raw vegetables such as carrots, celery, broccoli, or cauliflower. Drink low-calorie soft drinks or try chewing sugarless gum if you need to have something in your mouth.

Limit the Amount of Food You Take In

For some, the type of food is not the problem; rather it is overeating all foods at mealtime. Large helpings as well as seconds or thirds can significantly tip the calorie balance in favor of overfat. If this is your problem, sticking to your menu plan and measuring all portions is helpful. Serve yourself on small plates to limit the size of your portion.

It is also helpful to have available a small scale to weigh your foods, and a measuring cup, spoons, and a ruler to ensure that you adhere to the portions and sizes your plan calls for. Perhaps you might even leave some food uneaten on your plate. Before your meal, fill up with water or low-calorie liquids. Eat slowly; take twenty minutes or longer to finish a meal. Put your utensils down in between bites. If there are leftovers, put them away quickly.

YOUR FITNESS PROFILE 8-5
A Personal Weight Control Contract

Objective: To draw up a personal contract for weight control.

Directions:

1. Review Table 1-2 in Chapter 1 to help you decide on the specific body composition goals you want to list in your contract.
2. Refer to Profile 8-1A or Profile 8-1B to determine your target weight, target date, and your weekly negative-calorie-balance goals.
3. Review Profiles 8-2, 8-3, and 8-4 to help you determine your calorie intake and output goals.
4. Consult the discussion on selecting a sport or activity (pp. 258–262) to help you decide on the physical activities that you want to commit yourself to in your contract. Once you have decided on specific activities, it is most useful to list the exercise intensity and duration as well as the specific days when you expect to participate in the activities.
5. Note the date you want to begin your program. Then sign your contract along with a witness, someone who can hold you accountable.

Weight Control Contract

I, _____ , am contracting with myself to follow a weight control program of exercise and diet management to help me alter my body composition.

The body composition goals that I expect to achieve are:

1. _____

2. _____

3. _____

4. _____

5. _____

I expect to achieve a target weight of _____ lbs. by the target date of _____ .

During this time, my weekly negative-calorie-balance goal is _____ calories.

My diet plan will include a daily food intake of _____ calories.

My exercise plan will include a daily output of _____ calories.

Physical Activity Plan

Activities*	Session duration	Frequency (Check √)						
		M.	Tu.	W.	Th.	F.	Sa.	Su.
1.								
2.								
3.								
4.								
5.								
6.								
7.								

I will begin my program on ⎯⎯⎯⎯⎯⎯⎯⎯⎯⎯ .

I agree to maintain a record of my progress, and, if necessary, revise my goals.

Signed ⎯⎯⎯⎯⎯⎯⎯⎯⎯⎯ Date ⎯⎯⎯⎯⎯⎯⎯⎯⎯⎯

Witnessed by ⎯⎯⎯⎯⎯⎯⎯⎯⎯⎯

*Conduct all activities at an intensity within the EBZ, although brisk walking and similar aerobic activities provide greatest calorie-burning effects as a result of durations of more than 30 minutes to over an hour, five times per week.

PROFILE 8-5

YOUR FITNESS PROFILE 8-6
Plan Your Weekly Menus

Objective: To devise a week's menus that maintain your nutritional balance and stay within your target calorie amounts.

Directions:

1. From Table 8-2, determine the portions of each food group that you are allowed, so you can meet your calorie intake goal. Table 8-2 shows allowable portions for calorie plans of 1,000, 1,200, 1,500, 1,800, and 2,100. See Table 8-3 to determine size of portion.

2. Select your specific foods from Appendix C, "Food Exchange Plan," and record them for each day of the week alongside the appropriate meal or snack. The beauty of the food exchange list is the limitless variety of menus that are possible.

3. Place the portion size alongside the listed food. You can obtain the portion size from Table 8-3, "Calories per Portion," or from Appendix C. It is important to adhere to the correct portion size; for example, if you prepare a three-ounce portion of meat, that would count as three meat exchanges.

Sample Daily Menu Planner

Date _____9/16/87_____   Calories per day _1,800_

Meal and Food Group		Portions	Menus
Breakfast	meat	1	½ grapefruit
	fat	1	1 poached egg
	bread	1	1 slice whole wheat toast, 1 tsp. diet margarine
	milk	0	tea or coffee
	veg.	0	
	fruit	1	
Snack	fat	0	1 glass skim milk
	bread	1	2 graham crackers
	milk	1	1 apple
	veg.	0	
	fruit	1	
Lunch	meat	2	4 oz. orange juice
	fat	1	2 oz. turkey on rye bread, tomato, lettuce,
	bread	2	and 1 tsp. mayonnaise
	milk	0	tea or coffee
	veg.	2	
	fruit	1	
Snack	fat	1	1 cup unflavored, low-fat yogurt
	bread	0	2 T. raisins
	milk	1	
	veg.	0	
	fruit	1	
Dinner	meat	4	4 oz. broiled flounder with ½ c. brown rice
	fat	2	½ c. broccoli, ½ c. carrots, sliced tomato
	bread	2	1 slice whole wheat bread with 1 tsp. margarine
	milk	0	¼ cantaloupe
	veg.	3	caffeine-free diet soda
	fruit	1	
Snack	fat	0	3 cups popcorn
	bread	1	celery
	milk	1	1 glass skim milk
	veg.	1	
	fruit	0	

Portions allowed each day: Meat _7_ Fat _5_ Bread _7_ Milk _3_ Veg. _6_ Fruit _5_

4. Study the partially filled-in weekly menu before using the blank worksheet. The example presents an 1,800-calorie plan. For variety, you may change the number of portions of various food groups.

Daily Menu Planner

Date _____   Calories per day _____

Meal and Food Group		Portions	Menus
Breakfast	meat fat bread milk veg. fruit		
Snack	fat bread milk veg. fruit		
Lunch	meat fat bread milk veg. fruit		
Snack	fat bread milk veg. fruit		
Dinner	meat fat bread milk veg. fruit		
Snack	fat bread milk veg. fruit		

Portions allowed each day: Meat _____ Fat _____ Bread _____ Milk _____ Veg. _____ Fruit _____

PROFILE 8-7

YOUR FITNESS PROFILE 8-7
Weight Control Progress Graph

Objective: To chart your weight control progress to keep you on track.

Directions:

1. Note your starting weight on the graph.
2. Draw a dot under each week alongside the appropriate weight change. Place each dot in the center of the appropriate box.
3. Connect the dots from week to week. This will provide a graphic picture of your progress. It is not uncommon for a temporary rise in weight to occur occasionally, but the general trend should be downward. If it is not, you may have to decrease your calorie intake or increase your calorie output through physical activity. The solid line shows a gradual weight loss of one pound per week. If your dots are located along the line, you are losing at the rate of one pound per week. Below the line you will be losing at a more rapid rate and above the line at a slower rate.

Weight Control Graph

Starting Weight: _____

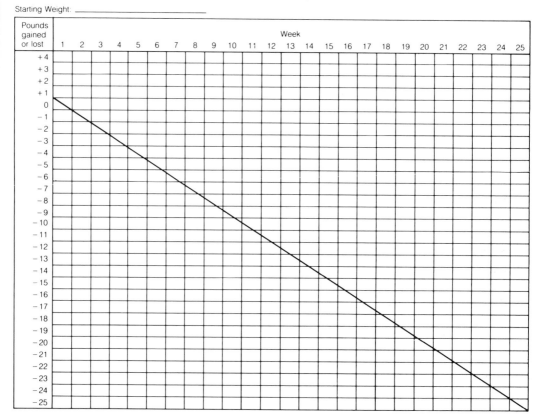

EXERCISE TIPS

1. Burn more calories routinely.
    a. No more elevators or escalators—use stairs only.
    b. Park at the end of parking lots—walk farther to your destinations.
    c. Do some sort of exercising while you watch TV.
    d. Whenever possible, walk instead of ride.
    e. Whenever possible, use manual tools and instruments instead of power tools.
    f. Pace instead of standing; stand instead of sitting; sit instead of lying down.
    g. During the work or school day, find a way to climb some stairs after every hour or two.
2. Plan regular exercise periods each day.
    a. Walking, jogging, cycling, cross-country skiing, rowing, and swimming are the big calorie burners. Hacky-sack seems like moderate aerobic dance; done for a long period, it will burn calories at the rate of moderate aerobic dance.
    b. The greater the duration of the activity, the more calories you will burn.
    c. Do some muscular strength and muscular endurance activity—more muscle means a higher basal metabolism. This means that you will burn more calories at all times, even while resting.
    d. Weights, weight machines, the exercise wheel, push-ups, sit-ups, and so on, all build muscle.

Change Environmental Cues That Trigger Eating

Eating while reading or watching TV or during class breaks often causes us to take in too many calories. Certain friends or relatives can be instrumental in coaxing us to eat more than we should. Events such as parties, holidays, or special celebrations all seem like good excuses to move away from our plans and good intentions. Being aware of these situations and either avoiding them or replacing the high-calorie eating with low-calorie snacks can help. Try to eat only in designated eating places. Avoid doing anything else while you eat. Tell people not to offer you food, and if you are going to a party, bring along your own low-calorie drinks.

Avoid Using Food to Replace Feelings

For some overeaters, emotions such as boredom, joy, anger, depression, or disappointment trigger the intake of food. These patterns develop over many years and require a conscious effort to change. Try to express your feelings more directly or find more constructive approaches for dealing with them.

Avoid Buying and Storing Troublesome Foods

If high-calorie foods are not around, they are less likely to create problems. If you do the shopping, do so only after you have eaten. Shop from a list, and cover stored foods in opaque wrapping to avoid temptation.

THINGS TO KEEP IN MIND

1. It is essential that you eat breakfast and all meals, including snacks, daily.

2. You are trying to become inefficient at storing body fat while at the same time becoming efficient at removing or burning body fat.

3. When you limit yourself to a few meals per day, your body responds by slowing your metabolism and thus improves its ability to conserve energy and store fat. This is the opposite of what you want to accomplish.

4. Whenever possible, walk after a meal to burn fat while it is still in the bloodstream and before it reaches the fat storage cells.

5. It takes the appetite control center about 20 minutes to receive the message that you have eaten enough. Therefore, eat slowly; use a teaspoon instead of a tablespoon; chew each mouthful of food ten or more times before swallowing; put the fork or spoon down between each mouthful.

6. Dieting without exercise usually leads to a lowered resting metabolism, which makes it harder and harder to lose fat by limiting your food.

7. Exercise raises the metabolism in three ways:
   a. It causes the body to require more calories during activity.
   b. It causes the burning of more calories at rest for some time after the actual exercise is over.
   c. It builds muscle, which burns more calories at rest than fat does.

8. This system for losing fat and thus reducing weight is specifically designed to be slow and gradual. It has a better chance for lasting success than any crash diet does. It changes or alters the habits that caused weight gain in the first place.

Make Wise Choices When Eating Out

You can minimize the high-calorie pitfalls often associated with eating out. Select restaurants that provide low-calorie alternatives. Avoid fried foods or those rich in gravies; order broiled or baked foods instead. Request that gravies and salad dressings be served on the side. Have the bread and butter removed from your table. Order skimmed milk or diet drinks or just stick to water. Avoid desserts. When you are invited to eat at a friend's or relative's home, let the host or hostess know about your efforts to lose weight.

THE ROAD TO SUCCESS

Losing weight and maintaining the loss as a permanent change in body composition are difficult to accomplish. If they were easy, there would not be a proliferation of books and programs, each professing to be the best way to achieve prompt and long-lasting weight loss. Nor would so many people try first one and then an endless series of other programs—weight is repeatedly lost, only to be regained each time.

The only road to potential success is complicated, requiring changes in the way you eat and in your approach to exercise. You can't expect to achieve permanent lifestyle changes overnight. If you are absolutely determined to control your weight, follow the seven-step program and stick with it. Once you begin to lose weight, your desire to continue will become automatic and you are sure to have significantly altered your daily habits with regard to food and exercise.

9

Managing Stress

After you've read this chapter, you will be able to:

Identify the temporary physiological changes triggered by stress.

Compute your personal stress score.

Recognize the early warning signs of distress.

Recognize the potential of exercise as a stress management technique.

Select stress management strategies and techniques that can best satisfy personal needs.

Experiment with selected relaxation techniques.

When one of our cave-dwelling ancestors was suddenly confronted by a saber-toothed tiger, his body automatically prepared for action. His heart pumped faster; he began to sweat; his blood pressure soared and adrenaline poured into his bloodstream; blood sugar increased; and muscles tensed. All this gave him an "edge," enabling him to fight—or to run away—more successfully. Once he had dealt with the danger and he could rest in safety, his body returned to its normal level of functioning. In 1914, Harvard physiologist Walter Cannon labeled this bodily response to threatening situations the "fight or flight" response. Not until forty years later, though, did Hans Selye of Canada popularize the word *stress* to describe this natural phenomenon. And only within the last few years have scientists begun to recognize the negative effects of recurring stress.

Despite vast differences between life in the stone age and in our civilized state, we continue to be plagued by problems resulting from stress. Today the saber-toothed tigers are most often situations, people, or events (called *stressors*) that seem to elicit the same "fight or flight" response our earliest ancestors experienced. Unfortunately, neither fighting nor fleeing is an acceptable, civilized response to these modern-day "tigers." Physical arousal in response to physical threat is usually brief and generally dissipated by immediate action. Suppression of the now-inappropriate physical reaction often leads to a build-up in the products of the body's stress response. We must, therefore, find new ways of coping with today's stressors. We need to learn how to reduce our stress response to manageable levels. In addition, we must learn to rid ourselves of accumulated stress and tension by mastering effective relaxation and coping skills, and then we must practice these skills daily.

It is important to note that stress is natural; a certain amount is useful in improving performance. The veteran stage actor and athlete could experience stress at a level that actually improves performance. The level of stress that induces good health and improved performance is known as *eustress*. When stress increases to a point at which health and performance suffer, it is best described as *distress*.

Modern-day saber-toothed tigers are still causing stress.

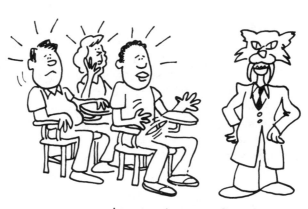

TODAY WE'RE HAVING A POP QUIZ.

FIGHT OR FLIGHT

Sudden and dramatic physiological changes take place to help you survive an extreme threat. These changes are designed to help you fight off the danger or escape from it:

- Your heart rate becomes faster, thus pumping blood more quickly. The faster pace meets your muscles' increased demands for oxygen and nutrients and also dissipates waste products more quickly.
- Your blood pressure rises with the increase in your heart rate.
- Your breathing becomes rapid and shallow.
- Hormones such as epinephrine (adrenaline) pour into your bloodstream.
- All your senses become more efficient.
- Your liver secretes sugar into your blood to meet increased energy needs.
- Your muscles become tense to enhance movement.
- The flow of blood increases to your muscles and brain.
- Blood flow to your digestive organs is restricted.
- Blood flow is slowed to your hands and feet as protection against excessive bleeding in case of injury.
- Your perspiration increases for improved cooling to overcome the heat generated by your increased metabolic rate.

RECOGNIZING DISTRESS

Your first step in coping with stress is to learn to recognize its onset. Not everybody signals the onset of stress in the same way; yet there are similarities. For example, the early signs of excess stress or distress generally appear as mood signs (being overexcited, worried, or rattled), internal signs (chills, light-headedness, feeling flushed, heart flutterings), and musculoskeletal signs (trembling hands, stammering, stiff neck, twitching). See Table 9-1 for some specific early-warning signs. By monitoring these early signs—especially your own particular pattern—you can avoid or confront more effectively the stressors that create problems for you. Continued stress can manifest itself in physical symptoms such as chronic diarrhea or constipation, headache, back pain, pounding heart, and skin rashes. (Before assuming that these symptoms are stress related, though, it is important to eliminate any purely medical cause.)

STRESSORS

It is natural to believe that a particular event, such as being corrected by your professor, is highly stressful. But some people welcome such an event. They perceive it

TABLE 9-1   Recognizing Distress

Mood signs

I feel "jumpy"
I have trouble sleeping at night
I worry
I respond with more anger than necessary
I feel insecure

Internal signs

My hands feel moist and cold
I sweat profusely
I feel my heart pounding
My stomach becomes upset

Musculoskeletal signs

My jaw muscles get tight
I have frequent headaches
My muscles feel tense
My neck becomes stiff
I develop twitches

SOURCE: Adapted from Daniel Girdano and George Everly, *Controlling Stress and Tension: A Holistic Approach* (Englewood Cliffs, N.J.: Prentice-Hall, 1979).

as part of a positive approach designed to help them improve their learning skills. (Of course, much depends on how the correction is offered.) What may be a stressor for you is not necessarily a stressor for someone else. Basically, the best way to recognize a personal stressor is to monitor your early-warning signs. What happens to you before, during, and after a particular event are your best clues. Most people experience some discomfort connected to stressful events. Real problems arise when discomfort is excessive and lasts for prolonged periods before and after an event and when you respond to an event inappropriately. This reaction is when the by-products of stress build up in your body. One approach to assessing the level of personal stress can be found in Table 9-2.

PHYSICAL ACTIVITY AND STRESS

Since the stress response is nature's way of preparing us to respond physically to impending threats, it follows that when we do not take physical action, added hormones in the blood, increased blood sugar, and various products of the aroused state of our bodies go unused. Because we face perceived threats several times a day without fighting or fleeing, these elevated levels of biochemicals continue to rise.

If someone accosts you on the street, whether you fight or run away, you have responded physically, and your response is appropriate. As a result you are likely to have used up the extra surge of hormones and sugar, and your increased muscle tension and blood-vessel changes will begin to return to normal levels. It is when the

TABLE 9-2   Student Stress Scale

The Student Stress Scale represents an adaptation of Holmes and Rahe's Life Events Scale. It has been modified to apply to college-age adults and should be considered as a rough indication of stress levels and health consequences for teaching purposes.

In the Student Stress Scale each event, such as beginning or ending school, is given a score that represents the amount of readjustment a person has to make in life as a result of the change. In some studies people with serious illnesses have been found to have high scores on similar scales. People with scores of 300 and higher have a high health risk. Subjects scoring between 150 and 300 points have about a 50–50 chance of serious health change within two years. Subjects scoring below 150 have a 1 in 3 chance of serious health change.

To determine *your* stress score, add up the number of points corresponding to the events you have experienced in the past six months or are likely to experience in the next six months.

	Past		Future			Past	Future
1. Death of a close family member	☐	100	☐	17. Increased workload at school	☐	37	☐
2. Death of a close friend	☐	73	☐	18. Outstanding personal achievement	☐	36	☐
3. Divorce between parents	☐	65	☐	19. First quarter/semester in college	☐	35	☐
4. Jail term	☐	63	☐	20. Change in living conditions	☐	31	☐
5. Major personal injury or illness	☐	63	☐	21. Serious argument with instructor	☐	30	☐
6. Marriage	☐	58	☐	22. Lower grades than expected	☐	29	☐
7. Fired from job	☐	50	☐	23. Change in sleeping habits	☐	29	☐
8. Failed important course	☐	47	☐	24. Change in social activities	☐	29	☐
9. Change in health of a family member	☐	45	☐	25. Change in eating habits	☐	28	☐
10. Pregnancy	☐	45	☐	26. Chronic car trouble	☐	26	☐
11. Sex problems	☐	44	☐	27. Change in number of family get-togethers	☐	26	☐
12. Serious argument with close friend	☐	40	☐	28. Too many missed classes	☐	25	☐
13. Change in financial status	☐	39	☐	29. Change of college	☐	24	☐
14. Change of major	☐	39	☐	30. Dropped more than one class	☐	23	☐
15. Trouble with parents	☐	39	☐	31. Minor traffic violations	☐	20	☐
16. New girl- or boyfriend	☐	38	☐	Total _____			

SOURCE: Adapted from T. H. Holmes and R. H. Rahe, The social readjustment rating scale, *Journal of Psychosomatic Research* 11:213, 1967.

stress response is provoked by events that are stressful but not life threatening, such as a term-paper deadline or a final examination, that problems begin. In fact, your chronic stress response may include some of the elements of the fight or flight response, but not necessarily all of them. A common example is the tension headache. Here the muscles of the neck, jaws, and face tense to prepare for action. When actual physical action doesn't release this tension, the contracted muscles go into spasm after a prolonged period. If we stop to rest and relax our muscles several times throughout the day, we can often prevent tension headaches and other such complaints. Some stress management practitioners liken this to the "cave time" available to our early ancestors who retired to their caves after safely returning from a life-threatening confrontation.

Since physical action isn't always possible in response to a perceived threat, we need to build in recreational physical activity on a regular basis. To be most beneficial, your activities should exclude those in which winning and competition are essential ingredients. The best activities are those that you can enjoy as play. This means not worrying about whether you can increase your distance or improve your skill. Exercise as play offers satisfaction, fulfillment, and sheer pleasure.

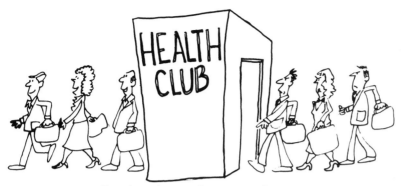

Exercise reduces and protects against stress.

When it is a regular part of your lifestyle, physical activity offers valuable benefits in stress protection. As a preventive measure, regular exercise conditions your body so that when stress occurs, recovery is more rapid. In addition, exercise enhances your feelings of self-assurance and well-being. Play, fun, laughter, and any potential elements of ego-devoid physical activity are all excellent stress fighters. As a treatment, exercise can burn up the biochemical by-products of stress and relieve excessive muscle tension.

DEALING WITH STRESS

There are a variety of strategies and techniques for dealing with stress. Table 9-3 contains a summary of five strategies. You may want to try one or more of them. Each method works well for some people and for some situations. Finding the ones that work for you may be a process of trial and error. Three specific techniques are described in greater detail for your experimentation—deep breathing, muscle relaxation, and meditative relaxation. If you do find a method that you think might work for you, you may want to do some additional reading or consult a mental health professional. It is essential to note that attempting to master relaxation skills is somewhat like learning to play tennis. It takes lots of practice and perseverance.

Deep Breathing

Although you can practice this exercise in a variety of positions, we recommend the following technique: Lie down on a blanket or rug on the floor. Place one pillow under your head and another under your knees. Bend your knees and move your feet about eight inches apart. Turn your toes slightly outward.

Scan your body for tension.

Place one hand on your abdomen and one hand on your chest.

Inhale slowly and deeply through your nose into your abdomen to push up your hand as much as feels comfortable. Your chest should move only a little and only with your abdomen. When you feel at ease with this step, smile slightly, inhale through

TABLE 9-3   Strategies and Techniques for Managing Stress

Strategy 1: Relaxation skills

a. Deep breathing: Slow rhythmic breathing to induce a relaxed state
b. Progressive muscle relaxation: Skill at recognizing the relaxed state and in inducing muscle relaxation
c. Meditative relaxation: Concentrating on words or objects to become relaxed

Strategy 2: Imagery

a. Relaxing through visualization: Imagining relaxing scenes that you can trigger in times of stress
b. Mental rehearsal: Mentally rehearsing a scene in which you cope effectively with a stressor
c. Stress inoculation: Mentally rehearsing a stressful scene that arouses a physiological response that is followed by your successfully controlling the response

Strategy 3: Planned coping

a. Anticipating situations that might cause you stress and implementing a concrete plan for preventing or reducing that stress

Strategy 4: Physical exercise

a. Planning at least 30 minutes a day of regular exercise, preferably aerobic activity

Strategy 5: Lifestyle change

a. Improving your health through adequate nutrition, rest, and exercise
b. Preventing or reducing stress by slowing down or learning to use your time more effectively
c. Developing supportive relationships such as by joining a group

your nose, and exhale through your mouth, making a quiet, relaxing, whooshing sound like the wind as you blow gently out. Your mouth, tongue, and jaw will be relaxed. Take long, slow, deep breaths that raise and lower your abdomen. The exhalation phase should take longer than the inhalation phase. Focus on the sound and feeling of breathing as you become more and more relaxed.

Continue deep breathing for five to ten minutes at a time, once or twice a day, for a couple of weeks. Then, if you like, extend this period to twenty minutes.

At the end of each deep-breathing session, take a little time to once more scan your body for tension. Compare the tension you feel at the conclusion of the exercise with that you experienced when you began.

When you become at ease with breathing into your abdomen, practice it during the day when you are sitting or standing. Concentrate on your abdomen moving up and down, the air moving in and out of your lungs, and the feelings of relaxation that deep breathing gives you.

When you have learned to relax by using deep breathing, practice it whenever you feel yourself getting tense.

Muscle Relaxation

The purpose of muscle-relaxation training is to learn to recognize the difference between muscle tension and relaxation. Once you master the technique of muscle relaxation, you will be able to relax tense muscles while you use other muscles to

TABLE 9-4   Muscle Relaxation Exercises

Muscles	Exercise	Tension area
1. Hands, wrists, forearms	Clench fists (as if squeezing a tennis ball); relax	Wrists, hands, and inside of forearms
2. Upper arms	Bend elbows and fingers to shoulders and tighten biceps; relax	Bicep muscles
3. Forehead	Raise eyebrows and wrinkle forehead; relax	Entire forehead
4. Eyes	Close eyes tightly; relax	Eyelids
5. Jaws	Clench teeth tightly; relax	Jaws
6. Tongue	Press tongue upward against roof of mouth; relax	Area around tongue
7. Mouth	Press lips tightly together; relax	Mouth, eyes, and cheeks
8. Neck	Press head backward; relax	Back of neck
	Press chin to chest; relax	Front of neck
9. Shoulders	Shrug shoulders toward ears and tighten; relax	Muscles between neck and shoulders
10. Chest	Press palms together in front of chest; relax	Muscles on front of chest
11. Abdomen	Raise head and tighten abdominal muscles; relax	Muscles on front of abdomen
12. Back	Arch your back; relax	Lower back
13. Thighs	Straighten knees and tighten thigh muscles; relax	Muscles on front of thighs
14. Lower legs	Point toes away from your head; relax	Calf muscles
15. Lower legs	Point toes toward your head; relax	Muscles around shins

complete a particular action. (It may help to tape this exercise and use the tape to guide you through your initial relaxation sessions.)

Sit or lie in a comfortable position with your eyes closed in a quiet room where you will not be disturbed. If you are seated, have your arms at your sides and your feet flat on the floor. Your head should be resting in a comfortable position. If you are lying down, put one pillow under your head and another under your knees (to prevent back strain). Have your legs slightly apart and allow your feet to turn out. Your arms should be at your sides in a natural, comfortable position.

Once you are in position, alternatively tense (tighten) a muscle, hold the tension for about five seconds, and then release the tension and enjoy the relaxation—a warm feeling—for twenty to thirty seconds. Repeat this pattern two additional times before you move on to another muscle group. Relaxation exercises for fifteen different muscle groups are described in Table 9-4.

A relaxation session should last about twenty minutes, and you should repeat each exercise three times. Eventually you will be able to relax your muscles readily and without working through each exercise.

After you have completed the exercises, remain in a relaxed state with easy, regular breathing. Yawn; then stretch and get up refreshed.

Meditative Relaxation

Sit quietly in a comfortable position with your eyes closed. Beginning at your feet and slowly progressing upward to your face, deeply relax your muscles.

Keep your muscles relaxed. Breathe through your nose. Become aware of your breathing. As you exhale, say the word "one" silently to yourself. Continue to breathe in ("one") . . . out ("one") . . . in ("one"), out ("one"), and so on.

Breathe easily and naturally and continue for fifteen to twenty minutes. If extraneous thoughts arise, simply set them aside and continue the breathing and counting pattern.

Follow this procedure once or twice a day.

It is essential that you keep stress at a reasonable level if you are to function well in school and at work and at the same time maintain a high level of wellness.

10

Choosing a
Fitness Facility

After you've read this chapter, you will be able to:

Apply criteria for choosing a commercial fitness facility.

Compensate for existing shortcomings in your facility of choice.

Choosing a fitness facility can be a complicated exercise in itself. A multitude of spas, centers, and programs based on every kind of physical fitness "system" exist today. There are the "no-sweat" path to fitness offered by some health clubs and so-called figure salons that focus on yoga-type stretching movements. Other facilities pattern their exercise programs on nonstrenuous dance exercise or gymnastic skills. Many provide sophisticated weight training equipment and emphasize muscular development. Still others offer a range of activities wide enough to include medically supervised programs to develop cardiorespiratory fitness.

Facilities with a balanced program emphasize instruction geared to the development of all five of the fitness components: cardiorespiratory endurance (CRE), body composition, muscular strength, muscular endurance, and flexibility. Some supply no-nonsense, balanced fitness programs that can get you in and out without wasting your time. Other programs, such as those conducted by community recreation departments, stress fun and recreation, with physical fitness treated almost like a side effect. Some combination racquet and health clubs and spas offer a variety of approaches. In addition, some large corporations provide employees with in-house fitness facilities.

The image of the gymnasium as a stark, sweat-scented space containing shabby and half-broken exercise equipment seems to be on the way out. The new image is one of attractive, shiny, sophisticated equipment, carpeted floors, mirrored walls, and other decorator-look appointments. Unfortunately, this classy image is sometimes marred by reports of shoddy business practices.

In August 1978, *Consumer Reports* noted "there are more than 3,000 health spas around the nation." Today there may be more than five times that number. They range from small exercise rooms and reducing salons to multimillion-dollar facilities with gymnasiums, swimming pools, running tracks, saunas, and whirlpools. Some spas are clearly consumer-oriented attempts to promote physical fitness, with such

NO SWEAT HEALTH CLUB

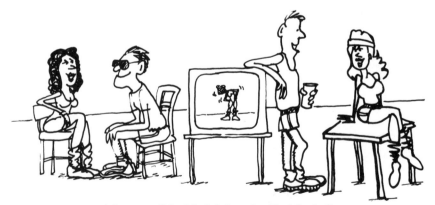

A "no sweat" health club is no health club at all.

204

fair business practices as pro rata refunds at any time. Others are barely one step ahead of the nearest district attorney. If the volume of complaints flowing into consumer agencies is any indication, many health spa customers are concluding that the only thing getting trimmed is their wallet.

People join health spas, gyms, or other organized programs for various reasons:

"I was most successful with my exercise program when I scheduled it after classes on specific days each week. I didn't spend a lot of money, but knowing I was wasting money I had spent if I didn't go to the activity gave me that extra push."

"I like class/group exercise. Peer pressure and sociability provide motivation after a week of hunching over textbooks and cramming for tests."

"I think that having a set time of the week and a special time of the day to do exercises, and especially having other students to do them with, really helps."

If you prefer an organized program—the kind commercial fitness centers or institutions offer—you should base your selection of one on answers to these questions.

Is the cost of membership within your means and the contract, if any, in your best interests?

If the cost of joining an organized exercise facility is going to be a drain on your pocketbook, don't join. Review the principles of exercise outlined in Chapter 2, and check the model programs in Chapter 7 and the sports and activities in Appendix B. Thus armed, you should be able to set up your own exercise program, which would certainly be less costly.

If cost is not a factor, shop around for the best deal, but measure the price against what you get in return. Be sure to find out about any extra charges for the use of courts or other special facilities or services. Another policy that affects cost is whether you are credited for enforced absences because of illness or vacation. Be suspicious of high-pressure selling and long-term contracts. Don't sign a contract until all your questions are answered.

Does the facility request appropriate medical information and, if necessary, medical clearance?

Some facilities require an exercise stress test and medical clearance after which they might also conduct a fitness evaluation (including a skinfold measurement to assess body fat). This information is then used to design an individualized program.

If the facility you're considering does not require medical clearance and other pertinent information, follow the guidelines outlined in Chapter 1. Whether you're asked or not, tell the staff about any medical problems you may have.

Is the staff qualified to provide exercise instruction?

If you want the best in fitness counseling, then you must be certain that those doing the counseling are fully qualified. Since qualified professionals receive salaries commensurate with their credentials, you should expect to pay more to a facility with such a staff. (Exceptions are nonprofit organizations such as the various "Y" associations, community centers, and recreation programs, and college or university programs.)

If none of the facilities you must choose among has a fully qualified staff but one of them otherwise meets your needs, then you can still manage if you take on the responsibility of designing your exercise program yourself by applying the principles of exercise presented in Chapter 2.

Does the facility offer opportunities for developing all five of the fitness components?

If you want a balanced program, you'll need either equipment or techniques that stress development of the cardiorespiratory and muscular systems. If a facility lacks such options as rowing machines, stationary bicycles, treadmills, or running space, then you may have difficulty in improving CRE. If resistance equipment is lacking, then you should not expect to develop your muscular strength and endurance to any great extent.

Exercise programs that stress "no sweat" and simple stretching movements can develop no more than flexibility. If you enjoy such limited programs, by all means participate. But be aware that you won't have a balanced program or one that will develop CRE. Even if the facility you plan to join does not have the resources to contribute to all five of the fitness components, it might have a professional staff that knows how to compensate for the gap. With circuit training or interval training and such exercises as aerobic dance, the facility can overcome the lack of some equipment.

Is the equipment sufficient so that waiting is unnecessary, even at peak hours?

An attractively decorated gym with shiny new equipment is all too often accepted as proof that the facility is adequately equipped. The only way to be certain, however, is to visit during peak hours. If people have to wait for a turn at the exercise equipment at those times, then the gym is overcrowded (or underequipped).

Some types of exercise programs require at least a minimum time at certain exercises (a stationary bicycle, for example) or performance of a circuit or interval training within specified target times. The value of such exercise programs may be impaired if you cannot get access to the equipment for sufficient time or at the appropriate time.

Are time limitations imposed?

Limited access is sometimes the result of overcrowding. But other time restrictions are sometimes built into the rules—alternate days for men and women, or "men only" and "women only" during certain hours, for instance. The times you can then attend might not fit in with your plans, so be sure to find out when the facility will be available to you before you commit yourself.

Is there a system for evaluating your progress?

A system for recording your progress is a necessity to provide progressive overload. Some programs provide individualized exercise cards that the participant

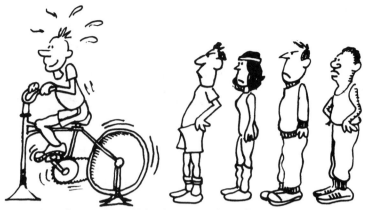

If possible, avoid facilities that are underequipped or overused.

uses during each visit. The system is more effective if a qualified instructor reviews the card on a regular basis so that adjustments in your program can be made as needed. If the facility does not provide progress cards but it meets your needs in other ways, be sure to set up your own record-keeping system (see Chapter 13).

Are enough instructors available to give you help when you need it?

If one of your reasons for considering a commercial or institutional facility is to receive guidance in achieving your fitness goals, then be sure that enough qualified instructors are available. Be aware that some "certification programs" are based on nothing more than a seminar or two. Such programs are no substitute for thorough professional preparation. Facilities can work differently: Some require you to make an appointment for assistance; others have instructors who circulate and offer suggestions on the spot or who check your progress card at regular intervals and offer advice. Whatever the system, be certain that you understand and can make full use of it. The system must be one that you will be comfortable with if it is to be effective for you.

Is the location convenient?

In addition to finding a facility that's open on the days and during the hours best suited to your schedule, it's important to choose one that is conveniently located. If you can find time during the day for exercise, choose a facility that's close to where you work. Or if early mornings or evenings are best, then try to find a facility close to your home or at a handy point between your home and your job.

If you work for a corporation that sponsors a fitness program, make use of it. Employee programs are usually adjuncts of the company's medical department. These programs are usually supervised by qualified professionals (physical educators with knowledge or experience in exercise physiology).

Are there enough activities to hold your interest over a period of time?

Some exercisers are so well disciplined that they can take regular exercise as though it were a measured dose of medicine. If you are one of these, then you should choose a facility that can provide a program consistent with the principles of exercise outlined in Chapter 2. If, however, you expect enjoyment along with your exercise, be certain that the available activities are the kind you like. If you like to try new sports and exercises, select a facility with a wide variety of activities to choose from. If other family members are to be involved in the program, then the scope of choices might have to be even broader.

Can the facility design a program for your special medical needs, if any?

A question to be resolved before you join an exercise facility is whether it can provide the necessary exercises you require should you have a particular health problem. There are specialized exercise programs, for instance, for cardiac rehabilitation, orthopedic problems, and other special physical needs. Most of these programs are associated with educational institutions, hospitals, medical centers, and the various "Y" associations. Occasionally, private clubs also offer these special services.

11

Programs for Special Needs

After you've read this chapter, you will be able to:

Recognize how exercise can be helpful in managing selected health problems.

Identify ways you can adapt physical activities to satisfy special needs.

Health limitations—whether permanent or temporary—are not necessarily a deterrent to exercise. Since the end of World War II, there has been wheelchair competition in basketball, and there are marathon competitors confined to wheelchairs. Skiers know of one-legged practitioners of the sport, and some baseball fans may remember Pete Gray, the one-armed major league outfielder who played for the old St. Louis Browns. Many blind athletes participate in sports such as golf, cross-country and Alpine skiing, wrestling, track, swimming, tandem bicycling, and rowing.

If you have been avoiding exercise because of health problems, perhaps such examples can get you to reconsider the possibility. We review ways to exercise despite disabilities or health limitations in this chapter. The suggestions we make about programs for special needs are intended as guidelines, not as models to follow in every detail. For one thing, people with certain diseases—arthritis, asthma, and diabetes, for example—require more or less continuous medical supervision and should not change their activity level or lifestyle without seeking medical advice. This chapter should not be considered a substitute for that. It's important for people with special health needs to keep in touch with their physician at regular intervals. But with a physician's advice, it's possible to freely adjust and adapt any of the exercise ideas in this chapter to meet particular needs.

HYPERTENSION

As many know only too well, hypertension (high blood pressure) is a common and potentially serious health problem. Although the causes of the disease remain unresolved, it can be controlled by diet, exercise, and medication. It would not be accurate to say that exercise alone can be used to treat hypertension.

There is fairly good evidence to indicate that with *moderate* hypertension, regular exercise over a long period of time has a tendency to decrease blood pressure, although that is certainly not guaranteed. People on blood pressure medication who plan to begin an exercise regimen should be sure to check with their doctor. The medication may have to be reduced in order to offset the effect of the training program. Of the exercise regimens likely to be prescribed, CRE programs seem the most appropriate. Increasing muscle strength can lower the blood pressure response to a given muscular load. However, excessive training loads can be dangerous to people with high blood pressure. Weight training, isometric exercise, and calisthenics can be risky; consult your physician before beginning such a program. An overall treatment program must be carried out under a physician's care, of course.

DIABETES

Diabetes mellitus is a chronic disorder of the metabolism of sugar, protein, and fat. It is due to a deficiency of insulin, a hormone made in the pancreas. If some combination of genetic, immune, and possibly viral factors makes your pancreas unable to produce insulin, you have Type 1, or insulin-dependent, diabetes. (The disease was formerly known as juvenile-onset diabetes, even though it can appear at any age.) Type 1 diabetics must take one or more injections of insulin every day. If insulin is withheld for any reason, diabetic ketoacidosis, coma, and death may occur in a few days. If too much insulin is taken, the consequences can be equally dangerous: Severe hypoglycemia (low blood sugar) can produce convulsions and coma.

Type 1 diabetics usually find that the more they exercise, the less insulin they require. Although the role of exercise in the balance between insulin and diet has long been recognized, the exact mechanism has only recently been explained. It now seems clear from studies in humans as well as in animals that exercising the muscles into which the insulin has been injected speeds its absorption into the bloodstream.

Exercise is not recommended unless the diabetic is under control. Diabetic control means predictably regulating blood sugar. If blood sugar is too high, exercise tends to make it go even higher, and the person risks going into diabetic coma because of the build-up of metabolic acids. If blood sugar is too low, then the person risks hypoglycemia (extremely low blood sugar) and may go into insulin shock. Diabetic control involves balancing insulin, energy intake (food), and energy expenditure (exercise). The diabetic who is taking insulin is involved in a daily and often hourly juggling act trying to balance these factors.

Injection site is important in diabetics who exercise. Injecting insulin in the skin over an active muscle, such as the legs in a jogger, may speed the absorption of insulin into the bloodstream and make blood sugar more difficult to predict. It is recommended that exercising diabetics inject the insulin over inactive muscle groups, such as the abdomen.

Only about 20 percent of diabetics can be classified as having Type 1. The rest have Type 2, or noninsulin-dependent, diabetes. Formerly known as maturity-onset or adult-onset diabetes, Type 2 is probably almost entirely genetic in origin. In these patients, the pancreas may produce normal or even above-normal amounts of insulin, yet blood sugar levels rise and the clinical condition known as diabetes follows, despite the seeming paradox of elevated blood levels of insulin. Type 2 diabetics lack sufficient insulin receptors on their body cells. These cell-surface receptors facilitate entry of glucose into the cell where it can be used effectively.

The beneficial effects of exercise are evident in the successful control of Type 2 diabetes. By exercising and also losing weight in the process, Type 2 diabetics—most of whom are obese—can increase the number of insulin receptors on their body cells and thus facilitate the action of their own insulin. When this occurs, blood sugar returns toward normal, and no oral medications are required.

If you have diabetes, you should consult your physician about suitable exercises. CRE should be the basis of your program, with activities chosen for their fitness benefits. But the ones selected should also be enjoyable for you so that you will get enough pleasure from the program to want to continue it.

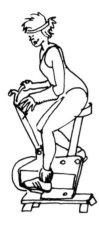

Injuries don't necessarily bar you from all physical activities.

ORTHOPEDIC PROBLEMS AND EXERCISES

There is a wide range of orthopedic problems—injuries and disabilities affecting the muscles, bones, and joints. Among the more common are muscle sprains and strains, fractured bones, torn cartilages, joint separations and dislocations, ruptured tendons, and tendinitis.

There is no substitute for competent medical care when such ailments occur. At some stage in your therapy, your doctor will probably prescribe reconditioning exercise. The exercise may substitute for surgery, follow the removal of a cast, or aim to recondition muscles and joints after surgery. A balanced program (to the extent permitted by the injury) is essential if you are to maintain and improve your fitness level. You may, of course, have to adapt your program considerably to protect the injured part. An injured wrist, for example, may mean you have to give up tennis. But you might be able to use a stationary bicycle or take up jogging. A leg injury may require exercise while seated or lying down. In any case, your program should include two aspects—general conditioning and a specific therapeutic exercise for the injured part.

Low-Back Pain

Probably the most common orthopedic complaint is low-back pain. Millions of Americans have suffered at least one episode of severe, prolonged pain in the small of the back. And a good number are under medical treatment for chronic low-back pain. The causes of all this suffering vary, but most authorities agree that exercise can help solve many back problems. And a few simple changes in routine body mechanics may also help. If you are susceptible to backaches, try one or more of the following suggestions:

- Avoid prolonged standing. If you must stand, support your weight mainly on your heels, with one or both knees slightly flexed.
- Walk with your toes pointed ahead.
- Avoid high-heeled shoes.
- Always sit with your lower back slightly rounded and with your feet flat on the floor—especially during prolonged sitting, as during a plane ride or auto trip. If this position isn't comfortable, try using a lumbar roll (a semi-firm cylindrical cushion). Place the roll just above your belt line after sitting as far back in your chair as possible. This method of sitting can produce the correct hollow in your lower back.
- Avoid lying flat on your stomach or back. If you must lie on your back, place a pillow under your knees. Lying curled on one side is usually the most comfortable position for people with low-back problems.

- To lift a load from the floor, squat with both knees bent and at least one foot flat on the floor. Keep your back arched. Always bend the knees. Never bend straight over from the waist. Never lift a load above your waist. Keep your hips and knees bent a little so that your lower back does not bear the weight of the load.

Four major muscle groups affect your back: the abdominal muscles, the muscles along the spine, the side muscles, and the muscles of the hips. The following exercise program will stretch and strengthen each of these muscle groups. Some people who suffer from low-back pain have also found aqua exercises to be helpful. Aqua exercises are either non–weight bearing or partially weight bearing, thus reducing stress on the back. The water is supportive and able to provide resistance in pain-free positions. Swimming is also a good choice for those with low-back problems.

Before undertaking an exercise program for the lower back, check with your doctor. And once you start exercising, you should keep at it. Always perform the exercises slowly and progress very gradually until you are able to do ten repetitions of each exercise. This process may take two to three weeks.

1. **Alternate knee-to-chest** (abdominals, hips, lower back)
   Bend one knee up to your chest; raise your head and try to touch your knee with your chin. Hold the bent leg with both hands behind the knee. Alternate first one leg and then the other.

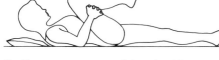

2. **Leg crossovers** (hips, back)
   Raise one leg and cross it over your body. Keep your upper back flat and your arms extended to the sides. Alternate first one leg and then the other. Turn only your hips.

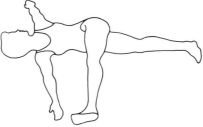

3. **Double knee-to-chest** (lower back)
   Bring both knees up to your chest. Curl your head toward your knees.

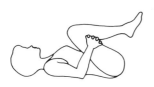 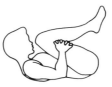

4. **Sit-up** (abdominals)
Cross your arms on your chest. If you use a slant board, start with your head at the high end of the board. As the sit-ups become easier, gradually lower the head of the board until you are doing sit-ups on a level surface. You can increase resistance by doing your sit-ups with your head at the lower end of the slant board. Always perform these exercises with your knees bent.

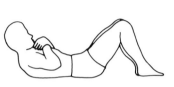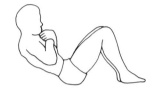

5. **Back extension** (lower back)
Raise your head and shoulders. Keep your legs straight and your hands behind your head.

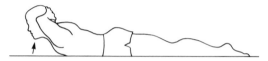

6. **Alternate hip extension** (buttocks, hamstrings, lower back)
Raise first one leg and then the other as high as possible. Keep your legs straight and your hands clasped behind your back.

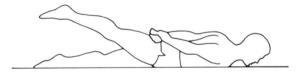

PREGNANCY

If you were exercising before your pregnancy, keep to your regular program, modifying it as your body tells you to. Always let your doctor know what your program consists of—the type of exercises, frequency, duration, etc. Or you may want to try the program below in place of your regular one. If you have not been exercising regularly before your pregnancy and you want to start, you must first get your doctor's approval.

The following program is especially designed for pregnant exercisers—both veteran exercisers and beginners:

• Warm up for five to ten minutes by walking—slow to brisk—while swinging your arms.

• Perform each of the twelve pregnancy exercises (see below) daily, as described. Do them slowly and rhythmically. Avoid strain and stop before you feel fatigued. They should take from fifteen to twenty minutes.

- Do the Kegel exercise (see below) to strengthen the pelvic floor.
- Select a CRE program from those recommended in Chapter 3 or choose one of the CRE model programs in Chapter 7. Always use your EBZ as your guide. If you have been relatively sedentary, the walking model program would be an excellent choice.
- Do not exceed a heart rate of 140–160 beats per minute, and the routine should be no longer than 25 minutes.

Recommended Exercise Heart Rates	
Age (yrs)	*Heart Rate (bpm)*
<20	140–160
20–29	135–155
30–39	130–150
>40	125–145

- Monitor your perception of effort while exercising. Effort should be no more than "somewhat hard."
- As a healthy sedentary woman you can begin an exercise program during pregnancy but you should not increase the intensity until the second trimester (months 3 to 6).
- Body composition is an important consideration during pregnancy. Too little or too much weight gain should be avoided. Work closely with your obstetrician to determine the ideal weight gain for you.

Kegel Exercise

The pelvic floor, which supports the pelvic organs, including the bladder, uterus, and rectum, requires strengthening to prevent urinary leakage and uterine prolapse. The Kegel exercise, practiced during and after pregnancy, is excellent for strengthening the pelvic floor. This exercise may make delivery less uncomfortable because it increases the ability to relax the sphincter muscles. Prenatal training of the pelvic floor muscles will make it easier to retrain these muscles after delivery. Alternately tighten and relax the sphincter muscles of the perineal area—the muscles that surround the vaginal and urethral sphincter in front and the anal sphincter at the rear. (Stopping the urinary stream several times while urinating will give you a good idea of what happens when the sphincters are tightened.)

As a very private exercise, it can be done (even when not urinating) wherever you are, and only you will know it. Do about five in a series, holding each contraction for about five seconds. Do at least fifty a day.

Pregnancy Exercises

The following series of twelve exercises takes about fifteen to twenty minutes to perform. You can do them daily, if you wish.

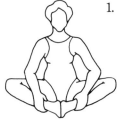

1. **Groin stretch** (helps make the delivery position more comfortable)
Start by holding your ankles with the soles of your feet touching each other. Lean forward and press your knees down with your elbows, feeling a gentle stretch in your groin and inner thighs. Hold the position for ten to thirty seconds. Repeat three times.

2. **Single knee tuck** (stretches lower back to help prevent or reduce back pain)
Start on your back with knees bent and the soles of your feet flat. Bring one knee to your chest, feeling a gentle stretch of the lower back. Relax the lower back as you hold for ten seconds. Switch knees and repeat the entire cycle three times.

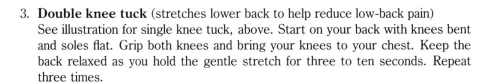

3. **Double knee tuck** (stretches lower back to help reduce low-back pain)
See illustration for single knee tuck, above. Start on your back with knees bent and soles flat. Grip both knees and bring your knees to your chest. Keep the back relaxed as you hold the gentle stretch for three to ten seconds. Repeat three times.

4. **Pelvic tilting on back** (to strengthen the abdominal muscles)
Start on your back with knees bent. Place one hand in the hollow of your back, the other on the rim of the hip. Slowly tighten the abdominal and buttock muscles by pushing down on your hand with the small of your back. Rock the baby back into the pelvic cradle as you roll your hips back gently. Breathe out as you contract the abdominal muscles. Hold the contraction for three to six seconds, then relax as you breathe in. Keep your back flat throughout. Repeat three to five times.

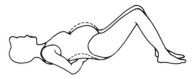

5. **Hamstring stretch** (to stretch the hamstring muscles)
Start with one leg straight, the other tucked in. Reach for the ankle of the extended leg, feeling the gentle stretch of the muscles in the back of the thigh. Hold the stretch for ten to thirty seconds. Switch legs and repeat the entire cycle three times.

6. **Sit-back** (for abdominal strength and endurance)
   Start in an upright sitting position. Reach forward with your arms and sit back to a 45° angle. Hold the V-like position for three to six seconds. Repeat three times.

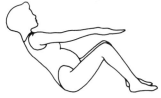

7. **Chest push** (for strength and endurance of the chest muscles)
   Start with your elbows bent and palms together. Press your palms firmly together so that you can feel the tightening of the pectoral muscles under the breasts. Hold the press for three to six seconds. Repeat three times.

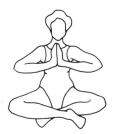

8. **Pelvic tilting on all fours** (to strengthen abdominal muscles)
   Start in a kneeling position with your arms extended for support. Pull your back and pelvis up into a catlike position. Hold for three to six seconds and relax to the starting position, but never let your spine sag. Repeat three times.

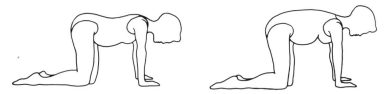

9. **Modified sit-up** (to strengthen abdominal muscles)
   Start flat on your back with knees bent. Tilt your pelvis up, flattening your back. Extend your arms and slowly curl up. Tuck your chin in and come up one vertebra at a time as you lift your head first and then your shoulders. Stop when you can see your heels and hold for three to six seconds before returning to the starting position. Repeat three times.

   Don't do this exercise if your abdominal muscles have separated (come to a point).

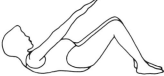

10. **Back arch** (to strengthen lower back muscles)
    Start on your back with knees bent and arms flat alongside. Do a pelvic tilt and then lift your tailbone, buttocks, and lower back from the floor. Hold this position for three to six seconds with your weight resting on your feet, arms, and shoulders. Return to starting position and repeat three times.

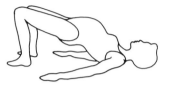

11. **Squat** (to strengthen thigh and hip muscles)
    If you have no knee problems, start with your feet flat on the floor, squatting half-way down. Hold for three to six seconds, then stand up. Eventually go into full squat. If necessary, have a partner hold your hands to assist with balance. Repeat three times. If you have knee problems, limit movement to half squat.

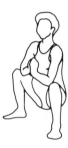

12. **Wall push-away** (for strength and endurance of the arms and shoulders and for flexibility of the Achilles tendon)
    Start supporting yourself with your arms extended against the wall. Bend your arms, allowing your head and upper body to slowly come toward the wall. Hold this position for ten seconds so that you can feel the stretch of your calves and Achilles tendon. Push away slowly to starting position. Repeat three times.

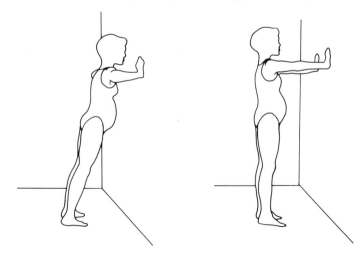

MANAGING ACUTE INJURIES: THE "RICE" PRINCIPLE

An acute injury, such as an ankle sprain or bruise, requires immediate attention if the injury is to heal quickly. After an injury, the tissue becomes inflamed. There is swelling and an increase in blood flow, and special blood cells and chemicals gather around the injured tissue. Healing is more rapid if inflammation can be minimized. The "RICE" method is the best way of dealing with an acute injury. RICE is an acronym for rest, ice, compression, and elevation.

When you get injured, rest. Don't keep exercising the injured joint or muscle. Put an ice pack on the injured tissue as soon as possible. If possible, compress the area with an elastic bandage. Finally, elevate the part to keep swelling to a minimum. Elevation lets gravity work for you rather than against you.

Nonsteroidal anti-inflammation drugs, such as Advil or Nuprin (available without a prescription), are also very good for combating inflammation. However, some people suffer from side effects when they use them. Check with your doctor if you have questions about these drugs.

It is always best to play it safe if you have an injury and you are not sure of its seriousness. If you have any doubts, have your physician evaluate the injury. Usually, sports injuries are minor, but some can develop into major problems if not evaluated and treated promptly.

12

Common Training Questions Answered

After you've read this chapter, you will be able to:

Recognize ways you can adjust to varied environmental conditions when exercising.

Recognize the effects of alcohol and cigarettes on your efforts to exercise.

Identify ways you can deal with common injuries and illnesses.

When you do exercise on your own—jogging, swimming, or weight training, for example—there are bound to be times when you wish you had a coach, trainer, or physician to advise you. You may only want reassurance or perhaps an evaluation of your progress. Some of your questions on specific aspects of training may have been answered already in earlier chapters. In this chapter are answers to questions that our students often ask us.

Is it safe to exercise outdoors in the cold?

With good judgment and the right clothing, most people can safely—and enjoyably—exercise even in subfreezing temperatures. People with heart conditions, however, should not do strenuous exercise outdoors in very cold weather without discussing it first with their physician. The average person will find that the body's heating system, like its cooling system, is very effective. When you run, you burn calories. This raises the temperature of the blood circulating through the body and thus warms the body. The hardest thing about exercising in cold weather is getting up the courage to go out the door. If you dress to keep heat from escaping, you may be surprised by how warm you'll be even on the coldest days.

Is there any harm in breathing freezing air into the lungs—especially through the mouth?

No, unless you're asthmatic. By the time the cold air gets to your lungs, it has had ample time to be warmed. Cold dry air may feel irritating to the throat, however, but you can avoid that by wearing a ski mask, wrapping a scarf around your face, or wearing a hooded sweat shirt and tightening the drawstrings so that the hood covers most of your face.

How can you prevent frostbite?

Frostbite is a condition in which body tissues are damaged or destroyed by freezing. The length of time you are exposed, the wind-chill factor, and how much moisture there is in the air and on the skin all affect your chances of getting frostbite. The most important element in prevention is proper clothing. The nose, ears, fingers, toes, cheeks, and penis are most vulnerable and should be carefully protected. The first sign of impending frostbite is a blotch of snow-white skin (usually on the nose or cheek). Covering the spot with a gloved hand for a short time will usually restore the circulation and color—no need for alarm at this point. Not to be ignored are later warning symptoms of numbness, tingling, and pain accompanied by a red, flushed appearance of the skin. Burning or itching may develop, and eventually the area becomes totally insensitive.

At this point, it's important to warm the injured tissue rapidly and gently by applying warm water (about 105°F). *Don't rub the skin with snow!* This folk remedy can be dangerous. Protect the injured area from further cold, and see a physician as soon as possible.

What should you wear when exercising in cold weather?

It depends on air temperature, wind speed, humidity, and the intensity of your exercise. An air temperature of 40°F on a calm day is one thing, but if there is an accompanying wind speed of 15 miles per hour, the effective temperature would be 22°F. So you must dress taking into account the wind-chill factor as well as the temperature. The intensity of your exercise is also important. The harder you work, the more calories you burn and the more heat your body produces. Activities such as running, bicycling, and cross-country skiing continuously burn a lot of calories. If you overdress for such activities, you will sweat excessively, and the chilling effect of your own perspiration may cause serious problems.

The trick is, of course, to dress in layers. The first layer should be nonirritating; a new alternative is polypropylene, which is believed to draw moisture away from the skin. Over tee shirt and running shorts can go a layer of dacron, polyester fleece, or wool, which are good insulators even when wet. Top it off with a tightly woven cotton windbreaker or a nylon one of a type that allows perspiration to filter to the outside. Hats and mittens (or gloves) are essential to prevent the loss of body heat. You can add or subtract many kinds of clothing depending on the weather. On long-distance outings (cross-country skiing, for example), you may need a small backpack to carry the extra layers as your body warms up and you begin to strip down or to carry warm clothing to put on when you stop to rest or in case of injury.

Is it all right to run in rain or snow?

Fine if you enjoy it. But keep a few precautions in mind. With most waterproof clothing, your body heat cannot easily escape and your perspiration cannot evaporate. Soon you may find sweat trickling down inside your clothes. Choose rainwear that "breathes," such as clothing made of Gore-Tex, a waterproofing product, or that has sufficient ventilation to allow air to circulate around your body and get through to the atmosphere. In snow or light rain, a water-repellent nylon sweat or warm-up suit will probably keep you dry enough. Be alert for icy patches and be prepared for the possibility of reduced traction. Obviously you should cut down on your usual speed when running in wet weather.

Is it true you burn more calories in cold weather than in moderate or warm weather?

Yes. Your body has to work harder to keep warm, and so you use more calories.

Can you acclimate yourself to exercising in the cold?

Apparently there is some evidence that people who exercise outdoors in winter adapt to the cold. One study indicated that after fourteen to sixteen hours of daily exposure for about two weeks, the study subjects felt considerably more comfortable in the cold, had warmer hands and feet, and shivered less than they did before. Fortunately, your respiratory system has the ability to warm even the coldest air, so you don't have to worry about your lungs freezing.

How do hot weather and high humidity affect exercisers?

In brief periods of strenuous activity, exercisers are little affected by extremes in temperature and humidity. But in prolonged vigorous exercise (such as jogging), they can be severely impaired. During hot weather, the circulatory system must divert significant quantities of blood to the skin, where heat is released in the form of

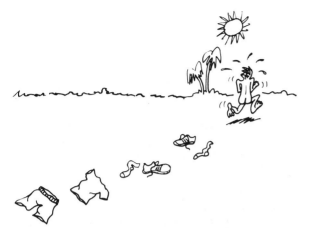

The most obvious adaptation to humidity is not necessarily the best.

sweat. As sweat evaporates, it cools both the skin and the blood circulating near the body surface. This cooled blood then continues to circulate, lowering the body temperature. Exercise makes a conflicting demand on the circulation. During activity to improve cardiorespiratory endurance, the circulatory system must deliver large quantities of oxygen to the muscles and continue to do so as long as the activity persists. These competing responsibilities of the circulatory system are further complicated by extremely high temperature and humidity. The hotter the weather, the more water the body loses in the form of sweat. And the more humid the weather, the less efficient the sweating mechanism is in lowering the body temperature, since evaporation takes place less rapidly when the air is already loaded with moisture. The combination of increased cardiorespiratory activity and loss of body fluid presents a number of health hazards to persons who exercise strenuously in hot humid weather.

How can one recognize and treat the different forms of heat disorders?

A person with mild *heat fatigue* feels extremely tired, has a rapid heart rate, and performs physical and mental tasks poorly. You can easily treat heat fatigue by having the person stop exercising and rest in a shady cool location, preferably one with a breeze.

Without treatment, heat fatigue may progress to *heat exhaustion,* during which the body temperature rises, blood pressure drops, pulse becomes rapid and weak, and sweating increases, which causes the skin to become cold and clammy. Persons with heat exhaustion look pale, may complain of headache, and may be mentally confused, vomit, or even lose consciousness. They should be made to lie down in a cool shady place and, if conscious and alert, drink plenty of fluids to replace the water lost by excessive sweating. It also helps to apply cool wet compresses and to fan them.

Heat cramps may result from loss of water and salt after prolonged exercise in hot weather. This too is easily remedied with rest and replacement of fluids and electrolytes.

The most extreme result of heat exposure is *heat stroke,* a medical emergency that requires the immediate attention of a physician. Heat stroke is a condition in which sweating is diminished or altogether absent, body temperature goes dangerously high, the skin appears hot, dry, and flushed, and respirations are deep and rapid. In heat stroke developed during exercise, the person may be sweating profusely. A person with heat stroke may be irritable or delirious, suffer convulsions, lose consciousness, and even die. Until the doctor arrives, make every effort to lower body temperature by using ice cubes, immersing in a tub of cold water, fanning, or applying cold wet compresses. Discontinue first aid as soon as the victim is awake and alert, but resume if body temperature rises again.

What is the best way to get used to exercising in hot weather?

Take four to ten days to adjust to higher temperatures. Weigh yourself daily when exercising in the heat. If you are steadily losing weight, you may becoming dehydrated and should drink more water. Reduce your workouts by 50 percent, and give yourself a chance to cool off at intervals, if necessary. Gradually build up to your previous intensity and duration. It is no indication of weakness to cut down your activity level at the beginning of a heat spell or after a sudden move to a hot climate: It takes time for your body to adjust. When you become acclimated to hot humid weather, you will not only sweat sooner and more profusely than you did before your body adjusted, but you will produce sweat with a lower concentration of salt. With your body temperature being regulated more efficiently, your heart rate will slow down to previously normal levels.

Is it harder for women to exercise in hot weather than it is for men?

No, despite some claims to the contrary. Men do seem to sweat more easily than women—that is, most men will begin to perspire before most women when performing a certain amount of exercise in an environment of a certain heat and humidity. This has led some authorities to conclude that men adapt to heat better than women. But other observers note that women can continue to work at a given intensity for a longer time in a given environment, and they conclude that women tolerate heat better than men. This point remains controversial. Conditioning can improve heat tolerance in both men and women. The more you work in warm environments, the more you become acclimated and the better your cooling system functions. Some people react to heat better than others, but there does not seem to be a consistent difference between men and women in this regard.

Isn't it harmful to drink water when exercising?

No. Water not only helps your performance, it also helps prevent serious heat disorders. During prolonged exercise in hot weather, you may sweat anywhere from one to three quarts of water per hour. You must replace that fluid if you are to continue sweating and keep your body temperature within normal limits. Dehydration may set in after as little as thirty minutes of vigorous activity, especially if you have spent a long time warming up beforehand. The American College of Sports Medicine recommends that water stations be placed at two- or two-and-one-half-mile intervals along a race course of ten miles or more. Another recommendation is that runners should have something to drink at ten- or fifteen-minute intervals throughout a long-distance run. In any case, you should certainly have something to drink after an hour of strenuous activity.

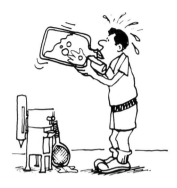

It's perfectly acceptable to drink as much water as you like during exercise.

It's a good idea to drink a glass or two of fluid ten or fifteen minutes *before* beginning exercise. But be careful not to drink too much too soon before starting, or a full bladder may make you uncomfortable.

At the end of a workout, you may find that you have lost a few pounds. The weight loss is entirely due to fluid loss; weight is usually gained back after exercise.

Isn't it harmful to drink cold liquids when overheated from exercising?

No. Studies do not support the widespread notion that drinking cold water causes stomach cramps or upsets the normal activity of the heart. Quite the contrary. There is evidence that cold fluids (45°F to 55°F) directly reduce internal body heat.

What are the rules for exercising in hot weather?

The following hot weather exercise guidelines may be helpful:

- Exercise in the early morning or late afternoon or evening, when ambient temperatures are lowest.
- Drink a glass or two of fluid ten or fifteen minutes before exercising. How much you drink should depend on the duration and intensity of your planned activity as well as on the availability of fluid during the activity.
- Avoid highly vigorous or competitive exercise in very warm weather—above 85°F, say, especially in humid weather.
- Slow down or stop any activity if you begin to feel uncomfortable. Symptoms such as dry mouth, hot head, dizziness, disorientation, or muscle weakness may indicate the onset of a heat disorder.
- Drink about one-half cup of fluid every ten or fifteen minutes during an activity that lasts more than fifty or sixty minutes—and even more frequently during high-intensity activity.
- Avoid taking salt pills or heavily salted food or drink before or during prolonged exercise. The body has its own defenses against excessive salt loss through sweating.
- Keep a record of your early morning body weight (after rising and urinating but before breakfast) to determine whether weight lost through sweating has been restored. Weight loss of no more than about 3 percent (or 4 to 5 pounds for a

150-pound individual) is normal, and most of this weight is restored within twenty-four hours after activity. Excessive weight loss or weight loss that lasts for extended periods of time may indicate a need to reduce or discontinue activity temporarily.

• Wear clothing that lets air circulate around the body. Avoid rubber suits, which prevent the rapid evaporation of sweat.

Is there any advantage to drinking fluids containing "mineral replacements" before, during, or after exercise?

Until recently, experts recommended cold water as the best fluid replacement beverage. However, now cold beverages containing small amounts of carbohydrate (about 7 percent) and electrolytes are thought to be best. Commercial products, such as Cytomax (Champion Nutrition), contain balanced formulas that satisfy the body's requirements for fluids, energy, and electrolytes. Drinking large amounts of fruit juice before and during exercise may cause gastrointestinal distress and is not recommended.

Is it wise to exercise when you feel sick?

It depends on whether you have a fever. Many authorities think exercising helps you feel better when you have a minor ailment, but most advise you to take it easy if you have a fever. If you do decide to exercise, it might be wise to reduce the intensity and duration of your workout. George Sheehan, M.D., a noted runner, advises that your resting pulse should be your guide if you are not sure you are well enough to exercise. If your heart rate is ten or more beats above your normal rate, you'd better omit your exercise session.

What precautions are necessary for exercising at high altitudes?

Exercising at altitudes up to about 6,500 feet gives most people little or no trouble at all. At altitudes higher than that, the oxygen content of the air eventually decreases to the point that the working muscles become deprived of the oxygen they need. In other words, the cardiorespiratory system must work harder at higher altitudes than at sea level. At above 8,000 feet, some people experience difficulty even without exercise. They have trouble sleeping or getting up in the morning, and they may feel light-headed and nauseous. But as usual, the body adapts to changes in the environment. The symptoms of altitude illness generally disappear within two to five days. If acute symptoms persist, your physician may want to prescribe a helpful medication. It takes time for acclimatization. If possible, ascend gradually, at a rate of one to three days for every 2,000 or 3,000 feet. Delay vigorous exercise until you are used to the altitude, and then begin at lower than usual intensity and duration, increasing gradually as you would when returning to an exercise program or beginning a new one. If you return to lower altitudes after an extended stay in the mountains, you may find that the training effect you have achieved at high altitudes makes it easier for you to work at the same intensity at lower altitudes.

What is cross-training?

Cross-training is practicing more than one form of exercise in your training routine. It became popular with the advent of triathlon competitions. Triathlons started out including swimming, running, and cycling. They have since been expanded to include combinations of many forms of exercise, including canoeing, rowing, cross-country skiing, mountain climbing, and horseback riding.

As discussed, the adaptation to exercise is extremely specific. It is unlikely you will be as good at many events as you would be concentrating on one. Most "cross-trainers" split their week so they are working on one type of exercise on one day and another form of exercise on another day. Some cross-training, such as weight training and endurance exercise, can actually interfere with each other. Studies have shown that it is more difficult to gain strength if you include vigorous endurance exercise in the routine. However, for most of us this is not a problem. You will develop some strength through weight training, even though you are participating in a jogging or swimming program at the same time. Scientists have only recently begun studying cross-training and triathlons, and much more remains to be learned.

What about foot placement in jogging and running?

For joggers and for runners at moderate speed, how the foot hits the ground can affect endurance and comfort. There is no question that a flat-footed strike or letting the heel hit first proves less tiring over a long distance than landing on the ball of the foot, as sprinters do. Runners who persist in routinely landing on the ball of the foot risk soreness from forcing the muscles to remain contracted over a long period of time.

Where are the best places to jog or run?

Joggers and runners are not as free as walkers in selecting a setting for exercise. Because the activity requires less intensity, walkers can usually get their exercise almost anywhere they choose. The simplest solution for a beginning runner faced with the problem of where to run is often the local high school outdoor track. Typically 440 yards, the track provides the beginner with a known distance so that performance can be measured and progress monitored. Some, however, may find that convenience and a smooth surface are not a sufficient counterbalance to the monotony of the track. Those who prefer a more varied setting risk twisted feet and ankles from irregular surfaces if they run on country roads or city sidewalks. Pavement, even if smooth, can be jarring to a runner over time. Indoor tracks that are banked provide a special hazard: Running on a concave surface will exert uneven force on each foot. If you reverse your direction every now and then, you may be able to avoid discomfort and possible injury. Do not choose a hilly area if you are a beginning runner.

What is the best type of clothing to wear while walking, jogging, or running outdoors?

Walkers can usually manage very nicely with any shoes that have adequate support. If readily available, hiking boots or shoes with thick soles and heels that provide good traction are ideal for walking. Regular walkers may want to consider investing in a pair of good quality walking shoes or training shoes used by joggers. Properly fitted, such shoes can make walking more pleasurable. Overdressing is a common mistake of the beginning walker. Avoid undue sweating by keeping clothes loose fitting and appropriate to the weather.

For joggers and runners, the proper footwear and clothing require careful consideration. In the very early stages of a jogging or running program, ordinary tennis shoes may suffice. To stick with sneakers over time, however, could lead to foot problems caused by inadequate support.

Even for the beginner, it pays to buy a pair of training shoes that fit well. But limit your selection to training shoes: The more delicate and light racing shoes are not for everyday use. Look for a lightweight shoe that's flexible, one that bends easily at the ball of the foot but is fairly rigid from the front of the arch to the heel. The shoe should provide cushioning that gradually thickens at the heel—to about twice the thickness of the front part of the shoe. That way the shoe will ease the stress on the heel as it strikes the ground. A firm heel counter helps keep the foot stable. The toe box should be comfortable, allowing for movement of the toes. Uppers should be soft. The best test of a shoe, no matter the price or its reputation, is how it fits you and how it works for you as a runner.

Not all runners use socks, but those who do usually prefer orlon socks. Nylon and cotton tend to retain heat and moisture, increasing the possibility of blisters. Calf-length tubes provide more protection in winter than ankle socks. For some runners, two pairs of socks help prevent blisters: first a lightweight cotton pair and then a thicker pair. Others find that two pairs of socks cramp the foot. A new alternative is socks made of polypropylene, which is supposed to let the perspiration escape and so keep your feet dry.

On a cool day, a sweat suit can be handy. The old gray model is just as functional as the sleek new warm-up suits—and a lot less costly. During the winter months, mittens will help retain body heat more than gloves. Some people, especially those tending to baldness or with very short hair, like to use a cap year-round. In winter, a cap provides warmth and in summer, protection from the heat of the sun. Ski caps in extremely cold weather are useful because they can double as face masks.

Cotton shorts and shirts absorb sweat more efficiently than nylon clothing, but you can launder nylon more easily. You can even take nylon shorts and a shirt into the shower and wash off the sweat as you soap up.

If you run after dark, wear reflectors so you will be visible to motorists.

What about jogging in a smoggy city?

Air pollution may make exercising uncomfortable and even dangerous at times. And some people question whether the risks of running where there is a high concentration of automobile traffic outweigh the benefits of the exercise itself. Of course, no one should exercise outdoors during a smog alert or when air quality is downright poor. People with asthma, angina, emphysema, or other cardiorespiratory difficulties should avoid outdoor exertion when the air quality is only fair or poor. At any time, you should let your body help you decide how hard and how long your workout should be, or whether you should be out there running or playing at all. Any sign of eye irritation or respiratory discomfort may indicate that the air quality is poor and that you would be better off indoors jumping rope or pedaling a stationary bike. If you must exercise outdoors in the smog, try to do it in the early morning or late evening, when lighter traffic, cooler temperatures, and lower humidity make the air quality better. Look for places to exercise away from heavy traffic, such as in parks, along riverbanks, or on

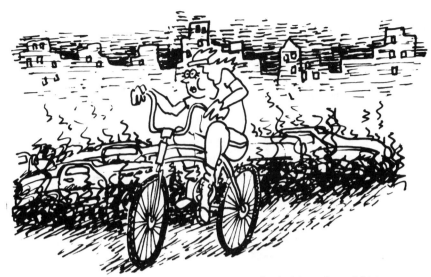

If possible, avoid exercising in air whose quality is fair or downright poor.

residential streets rather than commercial or industrial thoroughfares. And if you must exercise alongside traffic, remember that pollution is lower where traffic keeps moving fast than where stop-and-go conditions increase exhaust fumes.

Does smoking affect exercise?

Cigarette smoking does indeed affect exercise. First, smoking constricts the bronchial tubes, the pathways through which oxygen and other gases enter and leave the body. This narrowing limits not only the amount of air your lungs can take in, but also the amount of carbon dioxide and other gases they can expel. Second, cigarette smoke contains carbon monoxide, a gas that can combine with the hemoglobin in red blood cells and take up space normally reserved for oxygen. The less oxygen your muscles get, the harder your cardiorespiratory system must work to try to supply it. Thus the more you smoke, the faster your heart beats. If you are a smoker, you can test this effect by taking your pulse both before and after you smoke a cigarette. You will probably note an increase of twelve to twenty beats per minute.

The immediate effects of smoking are only part of the problem. The lungs of chronic smokers lose some of the ability to process oxygen efficiently. Even without overt disease, smokers, on average, score lower in endurance performance than nonsmokers as a group. And after training, smokers do not improve as much as nonsmokers.

Can exercise help a smoker kick the habit?

Many people—including many former smokers—think it can. The withdrawal symptoms you may experience when you give up smoking are, in many respects, the opposite of what exercisers often experience on a fitness program. Giving up a heavy tobacco habit may make you nervous, anxious, lethargic, and prone to headaches. Exercisers, however, often say that they feel more relaxed, confident, and energetic and that they have fewer headaches. In this view, therefore, the good effects of exercise may provide some sort of symptomatic protection against the bad effects of nicotine withdrawal. There is no evidence, however, that physical training has any direct physiological effect on tobacco dependence. Certainly, many people feel that the investment they make in an exercise program can act as additional motivation to reinforce their effort to stop smoking.

What causes a stitch in the side, and what can you do about it?

The stitch in the side—the bane of many an athlete's existence—is a sharp pain at the bottom or side of the rib cage, usually on the right side. There are many possible explanations, but no one is absolutely sure what causes it. Some people think it results from spasms of the diaphragm. Others think side stitches are spasms of the abdominal muscles. One way to deal with this type of side stitch is to slow down or even stop exercising and push your fingertips into the pain site, while bending forward and exhaling. When the stitch occurs, breathe so that you thrust your abdomen out as you inhale. In general, try to strengthen your diaphragm and abdominal muscles by increasing your cardiorespiratory activity and also by doing bent-knee sit-ups. You might also try lying on your back with your legs raised, supporting your hips with your hands and keeping your legs moving ("riding a bicycle").

Some stitches seem to come from eating just before exercise. The theory goes that the blood supply is diverted from the intestinal tract to the exercising muscles, thus causing intestinal cramps. The obvious solution for this is to avoid eating for three hours prior to exercising. Still another theory is that gas in the lower intestinal tract causes stitches.

As usual when there are many "cures" for a problem, there is no single reliable solution. Take your pick and use whatever works best for you.

What can you do about blisters?

A blister is a small pocket of fluid that accumulates just under the surface of the skin as a result of heat, friction, or irritation. Blisters frequently appear on the feet, particularly if shoes are too loose or if socks get wet. Prevent foot blisters by wearing clean, dry, well-fitting socks and shoes that fit securely over the socks. The best way to treat blisters is to puncture them and let the fluid drain out. (Be sure your hands and the area around the blister are thoroughly clean.) Sterilize a needle by holding it in a flame until it turns red. Puncture the blister at several points around the edge and allow the fluid to drain; if necessary, press on the blister with a bit of sterile gauze to force the fluid out. Do not remove the skin from the blister. Cover the blister with a dry, sterile dressing of "nonstickable" gauze. Keep it clean, and change the dressing as necessary. Often it is possible to resume exercising immediately, as long as the bandage is tight and secure enough to stay in place and protect the wound. Consult a physician at the first sign of infection.

To prevent blisters, be sure to wear the right sort of shoes for your exercise, and be sure they fit correctly. Apply petroleum jelly to any irritated area as soon as you notice it. Avoid long periods of exercise with new shoes. Take time to break in a new pair. Try a ready-made blister-proof insole. Avoid exercising in wet shoes and socks. If you are a golfer or racquet sport enthusiast, avoid blisters on your hands by wearing gloves and keeping your hands and the grip dry. With new shoes or new equipment or a new season, take time to let your body develop calluses to protect potential points of irritation.

What can a person do about skin irritation caused by clothing rubbing against the skin during exercise?

The most common sites for exercise irritation are the armpits, crotch, thighs, and nipples. Liberal applications of petroleum jelly or similar substances may be helpful in both preventing and treating it.

How can you treat athlete's foot and "jock itch"?

A good preventive measure for both "jock itch" and athlete's foot is to keep the vulnerable areas dry with talcum powder and by wearing dry, clean underclothing and socks. The powder absorbs sweat, which encourages fungal growth. If attention to hygiene doesn't help, try over-the-counter products containing either undecylenic acid or tolnaftate. Both are safe and effective antifungal remedies. If the infection persists, check with your physician or consult a podiatrist.

What can you do about a painful heel?

It depends on the cause. Achilles tendinitis (inflammation of the Achilles tendon) is a condition many joggers experience. The symptoms can vary from mild discomfort following exercise to total inability to walk without severe pain. The Achilles tendon, which makes it possible to stand on one's toes, connects the calf muscle to the heel bone. Since it is richly supplied with nerve endings, it becomes very painful when inflamed. Tendinitis is most often caused by overuse. Moderate stress on a tendon may result in microscopic tears. With greater stress, the tendon may rupture or break entirely, requiring surgical repair.

Ideally, tendinitis should be treated with rest. Discontinue jogging, cut down on walking, and try to stay off the foot as much as possible. But go on stretching out your heels and ankles gently every day. You can continue to maintain fitness by substituting swimming or bicycling for the duration. When you feel well enough to resume running, begin at a reduced intensity, duration, and frequency. Gradually build up your exercise program, if there is no recurrence of your tendon problem.

If the condition is mild enough to allow you to continue running, you should reduce the intensity, duration, and frequency. Joggers, for instance, can alternate running with walking as a temporary measure. Be sure to stretch well and warm up thoroughly. (See the stretching model program in Chapter 7.)

Some people find it helpful to apply heat to the calf before stretching or to massage it with ice afterward. Check your running shoes. Running in shoes with badly rundown heels can cause tendinitis. Try wearing shoes with built-up heels to reduce the strain, or try putting felt heel pads in your shoes.

If you're a beginning jogger, you can try to prevent tendon problems by keeping off hard surfaces, if possible, until you have developed good flexibility of the legs and until you are sure you have the best possible footwear and heel padding. Be sure you are running so that your heel strikes the ground first (or at least the whole foot). Never run so that your full weight is on the ball of the foot.

To strengthen the antagonistic muscles—those muscles around the shin that work in opposition to the calf muscles—try walking on your heels or raising your foot toward your shin while pressing down on your toes, for example. There is a tendency among runners to ignore the shin muscles while the calf muscles become very strong. The result is an imbalance that can complicate the problem of tendinitis. A series of simple strengthening exercises can help balance out the musculature of the lower leg and foot and thus help prevent future episodes of pain.

If the problem persists, you may want to consult an orthopedist, a podiatrist, or a physical therapist specializing in sports injuries. Be sure that such a person has had experience with this sort of condition. Some people have legs and feet that simply cannot stand up to the punishment that running demands. If you are one of them, choose another form of cardiorespiratory endurance (CRE) training from CRE activities described in Chapter 3 or in Chapter 7.

What causes "runner's knee," and what can you do for it?

Pain under the patella (kneecap)—variously called backpacker's, runner's, tennis, or jumper's knee—occurs when the patella does not ride in its proper groove as it moves over the knee joint. The friction may wear down the underside of the patella, causing inflammation and pain. Several abnormalities of gait can contribute to this problem. If, while running, your weight tends persistently to fall on the inside of your foot—a position called pronation—the turning and twisting of the leg bones may gradually make the patella unstable. Twisting may be the result of running on hard uneven surfaces or of running in shoes that have worn down unevenly around the heels. The relative weakness of the quadriceps muscles (on the front of the thighs) compared with the strength of the hamstring muscles (on the back of the thighs) creates an imbalance that affects the pull of the muscles on the patella, thus irritating the joint. Less frequently, a runner with legs of unequal length may develop pelvic tilting that, again, may result in twisting of the knee.

If you suffer from runner's knee, try applying ice to the painful area as soon as possible after exercising. To correct some of the underlying difficulties, do exercises to strengthen the quadriceps and to stretch the hamstrings (refer to Chapter 7). Be sure you use good, well-fitting shoes with a solid shank and an adequate supporting heel counter. If the problem persists, consult an orthopedist or a podiatrist.

Sometimes the pain of runner's knee is so severe that you should keep all weight off the affected leg and give it a period of rest. Try switching to swimming or cycling until you can return to running, hiking, or tennis again.

What causes "tennis elbow," and what can you do for it?

Tennis elbow can be disabling. An inflammation of tendons linking the forearm muscles to the elbow, it is caused by an overload of pressure on the forearm muscle groups that results in straining of the tendons at the elbow. While the problem is called tennis elbow, probably because it is so common among tennis players, it occurs in all racquet, wall, and net sports (as well as among gardeners, carpenters, lumberjacks, and housecleaners). Authorities have identified the following as contributing to tennis elbow: using the forearm as the source of power rather than body weight transferred from the shoulder; hitting a ball off-center on a racquet; using a racquet that is too heavy, has too large a grip, or has too much tension on the strings; playing on a surface that produces a greater velocity to the ball and results in a greater force being transmitted to the forearm and elbow. Treatment of tennis elbow may require medical attention. Start a program to increase the strength, endurance, and flexibility of the arm and shoulder after the pain subsides.

As a preventive measure, try improving your stroking ability to make contact with the ball properly—by using body weight coming from the shoulder as the source of power. A two-handed grip to hit a backhand can also be useful. Proper warm-up, particularly easy stretching of the elbow and its surrounding tissue, is essential.

What are shinsplints, and what can you do about them?

Shinsplints is a term used for a variety of conditions that produce pain along the front of the lower leg, that is, over the shinbone (tibia). It is often caused by an imbalance between a strengthened and shortened calf muscle and a comparatively weak shin muscle—a frequent result of prolonged strenuous running or jumping, particularly on hard surfaces. The pain itself may be the result of microscopic stress fractures of the tibia, a reduced blood supply to the muscles attached to the tibia, or damage from overstretching or overloading the muscles and tendons surrounding the tibia.

The best way to relieve the pain of shinsplints is to rest with the leg elevated and apply an ice pack to the painful area. To improve the condition, try wearing shoes with a raised heel or extra padding to absorb shock. Avoid exercising on hard surfaces. To strengthen the shin muscles and to stretch the calf muscles, do these exercises: Raise up on your toes, lower, and repeat; bring your toes toward your knees against some resistance such as a weight; stand and raise only your toes (by standing on your heels). Reduce the intensity and duration of your activity, and avoid running uphill until the condition improves. If these measures fail, consult an orthopedist, a podiatrist, or a physical therapist who is familiar with runners' problems. You may need to have an orthotic designed and molded especially to fit into your shoe to correct your gait.

What are stress fractures?

Stress fractures are hairline cracks in a bone. They occur most commonly in the bones of the lower leg and foot. The pain of a stress fracture is similar to that of shinsplints, except that it is much more sharply localized. Diagnosis is usually confirmed by X-ray, although sometimes a stress fracture shows up only some weeks after it has occurred, when callus formation becomes visible. You may be able to continue exercising with a stress fracture, but at reduced levels of intensity and duration. In more severe cases, you may have to stay off your feet entirely for several weeks. To prevent recurrence, do exercises for the foot and ankle. If stress fractures persist, you may need to consider changing to an activity that requires less impact on your feet, such as swimming or cycling.

What can you do about sprained ankles?

A sprained ankle is a common complaint, especially among joggers and runners. A sprain is an injury to the ligaments that surround a joint and help keep it stable. It may be a slight stretching of the ligaments or it may consist of a number of small tears. If you don't give the ligaments enough time to heal completely before you resume your activity, your ankle may be susceptible to further injury. The best way to treat a sprain is to elevate it and apply ice as soon as possible. You may use an elastic bandage for support—psychological as well as physical—and a cane or crutches if the pain is severe. When the pain subsides and any swelling has gone down, you may begin to rehabilitate the ankle. When you return to your regular exercise program, be sure to protect your weak ankle until it gets stronger. Your shoes should fit well and have well-cushioned soles. Avoid running on uneven surfaces. Above all, watch out for potholes, roots, stones, curbs, and other stumbling blocks.

Does jogging only on Saturdays and Sundays do more harm than good?

Although weekend jogging does not satisfy the recommended three days a week of CRE exercise (see Chapter 3), it can, of course, do some good. If you jog regularly every weekend, you will experience some improvement in CRE. The only way it can harm you is if you try to make up for lost time by working out too strenuously on Saturdays and Sundays. Keep the intensity of your run within your exercise benefit zone, and keep the duration within comfortable bounds. If you don't push yourself too close to the limits of your muscular and skeletal systems, you should be able to avoid pain and injury.

Take it slow if you're only a weekend jogger.

How do you maintain fitness once you achieve your goals?

Once you achieve the fitness goals you've set for yourself, you can then set higher ones, or decide to go on a maintenance program to keep yourself at goal levels. Generally, maintenance requires somewhat less effort. You can reduce frequency, but you should stick with the same intensity and duration. Continue to keep your progress chart, however. If you begin to notice a drop in fitness, you should increase intensity, duration, and frequency to return to goal levels.

Does sexual intercourse take away from athletic performance?

Not at all. The notion that athletes would be well advised to keep away from all sexual activity while in training and certainly before an event is pure myth. Any moderately conditioned individual should recover very quickly from burning the limited number of calories used in intercourse (ranging from as few as it takes to wash or dress to, at most, a brisk walk). In fact, orgasm induces a state of relaxation and for some a desire to rest or sleep. This should not be confused with fatigue. Some athletes report that sexual activity helps to relieve some of the unproductive tension often experienced before an athletic event.

Do physically fit people have a better sex life than other people?

No one knows. There is, however, no shortage of theory on this subject. No one has done a carefully controlled study to determine if there is a measurable, consistent relationship between physical fitness and sex life. Many people who exercise regularly, however, do report that increased enjoyment of sexual activity is a major benefit of their athletic activity.

Do people become addicted to exercise?

Some exercisers, particularly runners, do seem to become addicted to the sport. They give their daily run top priority, convinced that they cannot survive without it. They run despite pain, illness, or injury, putting their all-consuming passion for the sport ahead of family, job, and health. Some runners may even suffer withdrawal symptoms if forced to stop running. They become anxious, irritable, or depressed; they may get tics, muscle spasms, loss of appetite, constipation, and insomnia. It is unclear, though, whether this extreme kind of dependency is based on physiological or psychological causes (or both).

What happens if you don't do any exercise at all?

After twenty-eight days in space, the three astronauts of *Skylab I* returned to earth so weak that they couldn't stand without support. Their physicians were alarmed, especially when the weakness persisted. The astronauts' cardiorespiratory fitness had evidently deteriorated during their four weeks of sedentary living outside the pull of the earth's gravity. Learning from that experience, planners at the National Aeronautics and Space Administration installed exercise equipment—a stationary bicycle in *Skylab II* and both a bike and a treadmill in *Skylab III*. As a result, the astronauts of *Skylabs II* and *III*, who remained in space two and three times as long as the men of *Skylab I*, returned to earth with very little loss of fitness.

Of course, the most sedentary person on earth has fewer problems than an astronaut in space, who does not have even the pull of gravity to work against. But an earthbound person who sits in a chair long enough may become capable of doing little else but sitting in a chair. Almost any physical effort would be exhausting for the totally sedentary person. Because the body adapts in time to whatever load is regularly placed upon it, the ability to work is reduced if the load lessens.

Is there a specific age when the body begins to go downhill?

Some physiological functions peak at the age of twenty, while others peak at thirty. It is difficult to know whether any physical decline is due to the effects of aging or whether it has to do with how inactive a person is. One thing is fairly clear, however: Older athletes do seem able to delay the aging process better than sedentary people do. Regular exercise that prevents the accumulation of excess fat and maintains high cardiorespiratory function can certainly help to protect a person from the so-called degenerative diseases of aging.

Is there an age beyond which training effects should no longer be expected?

No. Age is no deterrent to the improvement of physical fitness. Although it's best to begin exercising young and continue throughout life, it is certainly better to begin exercising late than not at all. A sound, regular exercise program begun late in life will not regain for you the level of fitness you may have had in your youth. Nor should you expect to achieve training benefits as rapidly as a younger person might. However, there is no question that your fitness levels will improve if you follow a sensible program.

Doesn't aerobic capacity inevitably decrease with age?

Yes. The maximum amount of oxygen you can utilize during strenuous work usually does decrease with age. But by following a sound CRE program (see Chapter 7), you can delay the decline and even improve your CRE.

What accounts for the differences in fitness and athletic ability between men and women?

It is obvious that the best male athletes run, swim, jump, and throw faster, higher, and farther than the best female athletes. Whether these differences in performance derive chiefly from biological superiority or are primarily the result of cultural differences and societal attitudes or both is open to debate. If you compare the strength, endurance, and body composition of large groups of male and female athletes, there are few actual differences between the fittest females and the fittest males. The range of difference is certainly wider within either sex than between the sexes.

Of course, there are inescapable biological differences between the sexes. Since girls tend to develop and mature more quickly than boys, they often outperform boys during childhood and adolescence. Once past adolescence, however, males tend to have a number of physical advantages over females. Males are generally taller, heavier, stronger, and faster. Their heart size and lung surface are usually greater, and their hemoglobin levels are higher; hence their cardiac output and aerobic capacity are greater, and their heart rate is generally slower. Their muscle mass is greater, so they are capable of generating more power. They have less body fat to supply with oxygen, so their cardiorespiratory system can deliver it more efficiently to the working muscles. Lastly, their shoulders are usually wider and their extremities longer in relation to trunk size, so they have a longer reach and stride than females. All of these generalizations, however, are based on averages: Within the normal physical ranges, there is, of course, a large area of overlap in which individual females outperform individual males.

There is also a marked difference in the way most families, schools, and communities encourage athletic participation for boys and girls from the earliest ages. High-caliber female performance has been limited by the amount of coaching time and effort women get, and by the quality and quantity of the facilities provided for them. Since both physical fitness and motor skills improve with conditioning, instruction, and practice, most women have been at a distinct disadvantage almost from birth when compared with men. Such circumstances, and the attitudes that bring them about, are changing in American society. Many parents are now equally comfortable giving their daughters sports equipment as they are giving them dolls or housekeeping equipment. And schools receiving government funds are required to provide equal opportunity to girls and boys in physical education classes and in after-school programs.

Can vigorous activity cause iron deficiency in women?

No. There is no evidence that exercise, no matter how vigorous, will deplete iron stores or cause iron-deficiency anemia in women who have an adequate diet.

Iron is required for the formation of hemoglobin, the substance in blood that transports oxygen to the cells. Dietary iron is found in meats (especially liver), fish, green leafy vegetables (not just spinach), beans, dried fruits, and whole wheat. It is more readily absorbed, however, from meats and fish than from vegetables and fruits. The body stores iron in the liver, spleen, and bone marrow. When blood is lost from the body and dietary intake is insufficient, then iron reserves become depleted and the production of red blood cells is impaired. The result is iron-deficiency anemia—the red cells become smaller, paler, and fewer than normal. With insufficient hemoglobin, the delivery of oxygen to the tissues becomes less efficient, and this, of course, decreases aerobic capacity and CRE.

Iron-deficiency anemia can place severe limits on a woman's fitness program. If your hemoglobin level is less than normal, you may tire easily and have great difficulty engaging in even mild exercise. No matter how regularly you work out, you may not be able to achieve the training effects you are striving for. If you find yourself in this sort of predicament, you should consult a physician.

Are contact sports such as hockey and soccer more dangerous for females?

No. Thus far no one has shown that females are physiologically more vulnerable to injury than males who already participate in contact sports. It is well known that there is a relatively high injury rate among males who engage in certain sports. The data for females, however, are limited. One study indicated that college women in sports such as basketball, field hockey, and lacrosse experience more injuries than women who play less hazardous sports such as tennis or softball. But these injuries are generally the same sprained ankles and knee injuries that are common among males. Injuries to breasts were the least common injuries. It appears that if women are given the same level of coaching, training, equipment, and practice time as men receive, they are no more likely to be injured in contact sports than men.

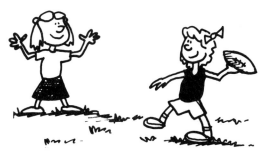

What effect will changing attitudes toward sex roles have on the athletic capabilities of women?

▓ Is it all right to continue a vigorous exercise program while menstruating?

Yes. No harm can come of it. The experience of menstruation varies greatly. For some women, it is accompanied by symptoms such as headache, backache, abdominal pain, and leg cramps. These symptoms should not create the impression that menstruation is a form of illness and that, as such, it is not advisable to exercise at that time. However, some women may not feel like exercising during menstruation, or at least during the first day or two when the menstrual discharge is usually heaviest and the discomfort, if any, is greatest. Many women experience little or no discomfort and thus rarely need to alter their exercise programs. Still others find that exercise helps reduce painful or uncomfortable symptoms of menstruation. In any case, there is no evidence that exercise during menstruation is unhealthy or that there is any unfavorable effect on the way women athletes perform if they compete during menstruation.

Women should exercise at whatever intensity and duration they feel comfortable with during their menstrual periods. The key is to listen to your body: It's an individual decision.

▓ Is it safe to go swimming while menstruating?

Yes. There is no evidence that either the exertion of swimming or the submersion in water (cold or heated) can harm a menstruating female.

▓ Is it true that exercise can cause cessation of menstrual cycles?

No. However, most women who engage in high-CRE activities, such as long-distance running or cross-country skiing, have very low percentages of body fat, often as low as 10 percent. There appears to be a relationship between a woman's percentage of body fat and ovulation and menstruation. Thus women who are severely underweight or malnourished and women who go on crash diets or who for some other reason experience a rapid loss of weight may cease to ovulate and menstruate. Stress may also be a factor among athletes who experience this condition (called *amenorrhea*). They have the psychological stress of high-level competition as well as the physiological stresses imposed by rigorous training and significant weight loss. Once the stress is relieved—for example, if the woman regains the lost weight or reduces her level of training—normal menstrual cycles usually resume. (Because there are other causes of amenorrhea, a woman should not assume that lack of periods is caused by exercise. An examination by a gynecologist would be prudent.)

▓ Can exercise such as jogging or rope skipping cause a woman's breasts to stretch or sag?

Exercise does not cause sagging or stretching of the breasts. Aging or multiple pregnancies are more likely causes. However, some women athletes report soreness and tenderness of the breasts. Some studies have suggested that a well-fitted bra can reduce such discomfort. Whether a woman wears a bra during exercise is a matter of personal comfort and preference, often dependent on breast size.

Will running enlarge a woman's calves and thighs?

Probably not. Like weight training, running need not develop bulky leg muscles. Women usually find that running burns up enough calories to reduce body fat, some of which may come off the hips and thighs. Running may also cause the leg muscles to become firmer and less flabby without necessarily becoming larger.

13

Getting Started and Keeping Going

After you've read this chapter, you will be able to:

List the goals that you wish to achieve through an exercise program.

Select activities designed to achieve your fitness goals.

Design a weekly program plan that notes your exercise intensity, duration, and frequency.

Sign a contractual commitment to a specific exercise program plan.

Identify steps to maximize program compliance.

Appreciate the value of recording program progress.

Even though you understand the theoretical basis of physical fitness, the importance of the five components, and the benefits you get from sports and other activities, you may still doubt your ability to stick with an exercise program. Perhaps you know from past experience or from your way of doing things that if you start an exercise program you may bog down, beg off, and finally quit. For those of you who are as likely to stop as you are to start, in this chapter, we offer suggestions to help you sustain your commitment to exercise.

We present five steps to help you get started on a fitness program—and to keep you going. Even if you think you're able to function well enough without a prescribed system, you may find all or some of these steps useful.

Step 1   Setting goals
Step 2   Selecting a sport or activity
Step 3   Making a commitment
Step 4   Beginning and maintaining your program
Step 5   Recording and assessing your progress

STEP 1: SETTING GOALS

What do you hope to get out of your exercise program? To reduce your blood pressure? To "get some exercise" because your doctor told you to? To become stronger? To improve your looks? Or do you just think it will make you feel better? Knowing the goals you hope to accomplish by exercising can be an important first step in a successful program because it establishes the direction you want to go in. If you can resolve why you're starting to exercise, it can help you to keep going.

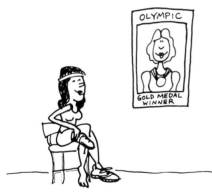

Role models can help keep you motivated.

Table 1-2 in Chapter 1 lists a wide variety of potential goals. Studies show that many of these are indeed achievable by regular systematic exercise. Others are more general, and the correlation between the benefits and exercise are often unproved. For example, a reduction in one's resting heart rate is easily and objectively measured and a predictable decrease can be a result of a cardiorespiratory endurance (CRE) program. Other goals, such as having more energy at the end of the day, are

241

more subjective and cannot be measured as readily. Even though some exercisers may not achieve all their goals, you will see their benefits.

In Chapter 1 we asked you to assess your current fitness level and determine which of the fitness components needed improvement. Then you identified the goals that you wish to achieve through exercise. If you have not yet set your goals, do so now as the first step in developing a personal program. Turn to the "Personal Fitness Contract" in Profile 13-1 and follow the directions.

STEP 2: SELECTING A SPORT OR ACTIVITY

The success of your exercise program could depend on the activity you select. A fitness program requires a commitment, and you are more likely to stick to it if you choose a program that is fun, interesting, convenient, within your means, and—most important—consistent with your health, skill, fitness level, and needs. The right program will enhance your ability and incentive to continue. Poor choices can provide obstacles or become drudgery—a chore you will eventually hate to do.

Table 1 in Appendix B summarizes the potential fitness benefits and other characteristics of the model programs noted in Chapter 7 as well as the sports and activities described in Appendix B. Select a number of sports and activities that appear to be the most likely candidates for your program. List your tentative selections in the activities column of Profile 13-1 and in Profile 13-2, "Your Program Log." Variety in your selections can help avoid boredom as well as let you put together a year-round program. For example, you may enjoy winter sports, but if your exercise is then limited to just a few months, your fitness level will also be limited unless you supplement your program with other activities. If your favorites are all outdoor activities, it may be wise to select some indoor alternatives for bad-weather days. Keep in mind that these are temporary selections. We suggest that you also take the following items into consideration when you consider activities for your program.

Fun and Interest

You are much more likely to continue an activity if you enjoy doing it. Start with what you are already doing and find pleasurable. Often, with some modification, you can integrate your current activities into your program.

Avoid pursuing a fitness program that you are less than fond of, because you may not stick with it. "Although I have jogged regularly from time to time," wrote Jan, "I find lots of excuses not to jog, so I guess I just don't like it." It is a good idea to undertake a trial period for a new activity. Before you make a commitment to a specific program, be sure it can hold your interest.

Your Goals and Fitness Needs

Most important is that your activities match goals and fitness needs. If you want, say, to improve your circulation, you need to select activities with high CRE benefits, such as aerobic dance, bicycling, jogging, rope skipping, swimming, or walking. To eliminate or reduce low-back pain, you need such activities as weight training and calisthenics to develop muscular strength, muscular endurance, and flexibility. If you're interested in overall improvement, then you should select activities in which you can develop all five fitness components.

To determine whether your activities will satisfy your goals and fitness needs, match the components checked for your activities with those checked for each of the goals. If the patterns are similar, you have probably made the right activity choices. However, if they don't match, you may have to change some activities to suit your body composition or CRE goals.

As you know, it is not the activity alone that determines whether you achieve the desired training effect, but rather the extent to which the program adheres to the training principles governing exercise intensity, duration, and frequency. We know that jogging has excellent potential to achieve CRE, but the potential is maximized when one jogs within the EBZ for a duration of at least fifteen to twenty minutes and at a frequency of three days per week. And if you added body composition goals, then it would be most productive to add at least another ten to fifteen minutes to the duration and two more days per week of activity.

To ensure that your program adheres to basic requirements, complete the columns in Profile 13-1, "Personal Fitness Contract," noting the intensity, duration, and frequency of each activity. You should show duration in minutes while you only need a check under the days of the week on which you expect to work out. It is expected that all activities designed to achieve CRE and body composition goals will be conducted within the EBZ, while the intensity of activities to achieve muscular development components will be designed to best achieve muscular strength, muscular endurance, or flexibility.

Health

Some people have health problems that direct them toward a specific group of sports or activities because they are beneficial or direct them away because they are contra-indicated. We have often had students come to us noting that they have back problems or suffer from diabetes or another chronic malady that they believe should exclude them from a physical activity program. In most cases, there are many exercise choices for them, choices that may enhance their ability to cope with their problem. (We covered a number of these problems in Chapter 11.)

Skill and Fitness

Occasionally, college students entering a fitness class express concern that they never had much athletic ability and perhaps it is futile to try. Peter recalled that he was in the "physical dumb group" throughout his early school years but regular participation in a carefully designed fitness program on a college campus led him to experience a gradual improvement in his body and fitness and to more positive feelings about himself.

PROFILE 13-1

YOUR FITNESS PROFILE 13-1
Personal Fitness Contract

Objective: To help you make a more lasting commitment to your physical fitness.

Directions:

1. Fill in the specific goals you would like to achieve.
2. Place a check under the fitness components you need to develop to achieve each goal you selected. See Table 1-2 in Chapter 1 for help with this step.
3. Fill in the activities you have selected.
4. For each of the activities that you have selected, place a check under each of the components that you can develop as a result of regular participation in these activities. Table 1 in Appendix B or Chapter 7 will help to guide you through this step.
5. Check off your intended frequency and indicate duration.
6. Sign and date your contract in the presence of a witness who can help you maintain your commitment.
7. Have your witness sign the contract as well.

Personal Fitness Contract

I, _Katie Price_, am contracting with myself to follow an exercise program to achieve and work at the following fitness goals and components.

Fitness Goals (Note as many as appropriate.)	CRE	BC	MS	ME	F
1. Prevent heart attack at an early age	✓				
2. Become more muscular; firm up		✓	✓	✓	
3. Prevent joint injury from athletics			✓		✓

Fitness Components (Check as appropriate.)

Program Plan

Activities	CRE*	BC*	MS	ME	F	Intensity	Duration	M.	Tu.	W.	Th.	F.	Sa.	Su.
1. Jogging	✓	✓		✓		140–170	30 m	✓		✓		✓		
2. Weight training			✓	✓	✓	8–15	3 sets	✓		✓		✓		
3. Stretching					✓	Mod.	10 secs.	✓		✓		✓		✓
4.														
5.														

Components (Check ✓)   Frequency (Check ✓)

Personal Fitness Contract

I, _____, am contracting with myself to follow an exercise program to achieve and work at the following fitness goals and components.

Fitness Goals (Note as many as appropriate.)	Fitness Components (Check as appropriate.)				
	CRE	BC	MS	ME	F
1. _____					
2. _____					
3. _____					
4. _____					
5. _____					
6. _____					
7. _____					
8. _____					

Program Plan

Activities	Components (Check √)					Intensity	Duration	Frequency (Check √)						
	CRE*	BC*	MS	ME	F			M.	Tu.	W.	Th.	F.	Sa.	Su.
1. _____														
2. _____														
3. _____														
4. _____														
5. _____														
6. _____														
7. _____														
8. _____														
9. _____														
10. _____														

I will begin my program on _____ .

I agree to maintain a record of my activity, assess my progress periodically, and, if necessary, revise my goals.

Signed _____ Date _____

Witness _____

*You should conduct activities for achieving CRE and body composition goals at an intensity within your EBZ.

So many sports and activities require a low or moderate level of skill that no one need feel unable to become fit. If you are not sure about the skill complexity of a particular activity, refer to Table 1 in Appendix B, where a special column rates activities in terms of the skill level needed to obtain fitness benefits.

It is true that some sports and activities require such high levels of skill that they are not a practical start-up choice for certain fitness-program beginners. You may not have the ability, time, or interest to become proficient enough in a sport or activity to use it as a vehicle for fitness. However, you can transfer many of the skills you have developed in past experiences with other sports or activities to seemingly new activities. This is particularly true with the racquet sports. The general skills involved in tennis are applicable to squash or racquetball. Similarly, those experienced with basketball, baseball, or football can transfer many of the skills connected with these sports to other activities such as the fast-growing sport of ultimate Frisbee.

Your current fitness level sets limits of its own. For example, if you have low CRE, it may be unwise to start a jogging program. A walking program could be a more appropriate way for you to begin exercising. Select activities that have an entry level that is right for you. Table 1 in Appendix B also has a column that rates activities in terms of the level of fitness needed before participation can lead to safe and productive results.

The way an activity is paced also determines the extent to which you can control its intensity. A self-paced activity such as walking or jogging allows you to determine how hard you would like to exercise and is ideal for someone who is sedentary. Most of the competitive sports are "other paced" and usually require some preconditioning. Some activities are a combination of being self-paced and other-paced. Table 1 in Appendix B has a column that can help you clarify how an activity is paced.

Age

In recent years we have experienced the influx of older students who are concerned that they may be too old to begin exercising again. Unless particular skills have been maintained over the years, it is best to avoid activities that require high levels of speed and movement, reaction time, and other qualities of motor ability. At the very least, it is wise to move into such participation gradually. Nevertheless, there are many fitness activities that older adults can participate in safely and with excellent results.

Time and Convenience

Time and convenience cover a multitude of factors. Special facilities are often needed, as is the case with swimming and tennis. Some activities are inconvenient because they may require trips to distant mountains, lakes, or oceans. Skiing and ice-skating are activities that require special weather conditions and are limited by their seasonal nature. The need for exercise partners in team sports often makes it difficult to depend on certain activities as staples for a fitness program. Time is also a limiting factor when you do not have the two to four hours required for an activity such as golf. Unless exercise fits easily into your daily schedule, it is less likely that you will continue your program.

Cost

Some sports and activities require equipment, fees, or membership investments that may strain your budget. Yet, there is no relationship between the fitness benefits of an activity and what it may cost. If money is an important consideration, limit your choice to activities that are inexpensive or even free. Remember that your selection may be temporary, so avoid a large financial investment until you're sure it's going to work out well.

Social Aspects

The social potential of a sport or an activity can be a double-edged sword. On the one hand, if other people are needed, you may have a problem whenever they are not available. On the other hand, having others available can be a powerful incentive to get started and keep going.

When you consider all these criteria and narrow your choices, you will find yourself establishing priorities and juggling the variables. You may end up selecting an activity because it's convenient and does what you want it to do within the time you have available, rather than because it's fun or interesting. Remember that selections are temporary, and you can experiment and change around. So, once again, try to avoid any large outlay of money until you are sure of your choices.

STEP 3: MAKING A COMMITMENT

To change your exercise behavior, you have to make a deal with yourself—not just count on good intentions. This time make a deal in the form of a written contract. The contract should clearly state what you are going to do, why you want to do it, when you're going to start, the specific goals you expect to achieve, and the specific time you set for meeting the goals. A carefully designed contract can help to convert your good intentions—and vague aspirations that encourage excuses and delays—to clear, detailed procedures that promote action. By putting it in writing, you make a firm commitment—and you may be more likely to carry through to your goal.

Profile 13-1, the "Personal Fitness Contract" you have already been working with, can serve as a contract to help you to make a more complete commitment. In the first step, you identified your fitness goals and the fitness components required to achieve these goals. In the next step, you developed your program plan. Now you have the opportunity to make a firmer deal with yourself by noting when you will begin your program and by signing the contract. In addition, it can be helpful to have your contract witnessed and signed by someone you feel could help you to be more accountable for your progress.

STEP 4: BEGINNING AND MAINTAINING YOUR PROGRAM

Always start out doing less than you think you can and progress slowly until you meet your goals. Give your body time to accept the change—something particularly important for sports and activities that require muscular adjustments. Don't let your initial enthusiasm trick you into exceeding your capacity. Be realistic, be patient—results take time.

The following guidelines may help you to get started and keep going:

Make your activity an unconditional part of your daily or weekly schedule. Set aside a regular time for exercise, and resist all efforts and temptations to deter you. Choose the time that fits your schedule, even though you may not always be at your best at that hour. Set aside *adequate* time: Allow for a proper ten-minute warm-up, a cool-down, and a shower (see the warm-up and cool-down exercises in Chapter 7).

Take advantage of whatever exercise opportunities present themselves: Walk to class, to the bus stop, up and down stairs—every chance you get.

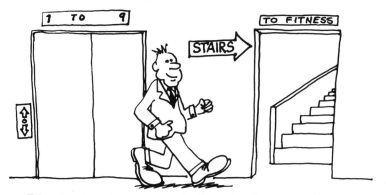

Take advantage of exercise opportunities when they present themselves.

Do what you can to avoid boredom. When you use a stationary bicycle or rowing machine at home, you might watch TV, listen to music, or read (with the help of a music stand). Some joggers use headphones to listen to music (but don't do it near automobile traffic—that could be dangerous). And you can do calisthenics at home to music.

Exercising with others can be useful, but try to keep the group to no more than three or four. Also try to form a group that shares your goals and is at your level of competence.

Vary the program. Change the activity periodically—alone or with a group. If walking, jogging, or bicycling, change the route or the distance every now and then.

Racquet sport enthusiasts might find it adds interest to change partners after a while or to try a new location.

Reward yourself for reaching minigoals. Until you achieve some of the goals that you have set for yourself, a system of self-rewards can improve your chances of sticking to a regular exercise program. For example, if you are on a weight training program, agree to give yourself a special treat—an entertainment or a particular purchase—when you have progressed to lifting a specific weight or a number of repetitions. Similarly, you could set mileage or time goals for such activities as jogging, swimming, or bicycling and reward yourself when you have achieved the goals. When selecting rewards, avoid those that could lead to backsliding (food, for example).

The rewards should be things that you enjoy and that are easily obtained. Some rewards can be expensive (a weekend vacation for sticking to your program plan for one month or special night out for completing one week), but don't go overboard; stick to rewards that are within your means. In fact, some rewards do not have to cost anything, such as sleeping late one morning or skipping a chore. Establish a hierarchy of rewards with small rewards for small steps and bigger rewards for greater achievements. You can do this by establishing a point system. You might give yourself a point for each day of activity with special bonuses at the end of each week or month. When you finally achieve 20, 30, 50, or 100 points, you can reward yourself accordingly.

STEP 5: RECORDING AND ASSESSING YOUR PROGRESS

Recording and assessing your progress after each exercise session—whether you make progress or not—can help you keep track of how you're doing. A record that notes the daily results of your program will give you a sense of accomplishment and remind you of your commitment.

Profile 13-2, "Your Program Log," can be used for this purpose. Also take a look at the sample progress chart in Profile 13-3 to get some ideas about how you might set up your own weekly record system. For a sample of a daily record system, see Table 7-10 in Chapter 7. No matter what form your record takes, keep it handy and post the results immediately after each exercise session.

If this strikes you as rigid, you're right. But remember that the main reason you're doing it is to help you get started and keep going. Stay with the record-keeping and give yourself enough time to begin to attain some goals. Once you've achieved your short-range goals, you'll discover less resistance to exercising—and a more favorable attitude toward the commitment to exercise.

There are no hard and fast rules to tell you how quickly you should progress. If you're doing a CRE activity, however, your heart rate can serve as your guide.

In the first few weeks, you may find that your program is unrealistic. If so, upgrade or downgrade the goals in your contract. If you find that your selection of activities has not been successful, switch to some other form of exercise. Expect this initial experience to be experimental, with many adjustments and changes.

YOUR FITNESS PROFILE 13-2
Your Program Log

Objective: To summarize your overall fitness plan and record your follow-through.

Directions:

1. List all the activities in your program. Include those you plan to do outside of class.
2. Post the date, at the top of each column, for each day that you exercise.
3. Make the appropriate notation for each exercise. For aerobic activities, note the total exercise time. For activities achieving muscular goals, simply place a check under the appropriate date. You should place specific notations for such programs as circuit training or weight training on separate progress cards in addition to checking them off on this chart.

PROGRAM LOG

Name _Katie Price_   Date 9/24

Exercise program	10/1	10/2	10/3	10/4	10/5													
1. Jogging	20 m	20	20															
2. Weight Training	✓	✓	✓															
3. Bicycling		30 m	35															
4. Swimming		15 m	15															

PROGRAM LOG

Name _____

Date _____

Exercise program

1.

2.

3.

4.

5.

6.

7.

8.

9.

10.

YOUR FITNESS PROFILE 13-3
A Weekly Log for Your CRE Progress

Objective: To record your exercise time or distance as a way of marking your progress.

Directions: Use this progress chart to record the distance you cover or the time you spend each day of the week on a CRE activity. (You will find the weekly calorie count in Table 7-4, p. 113.) You can use this log to record progress for more than one activity.

CRE Progress Chart

| Week | Activities | Daily distance or time | | | | | | | Weekly distance or time | Weekly calorie cost |
		Mon.	Tues.	Wed.	Thur.	Fri.	Sat.	Sun.		
1	Walking	30 min.		30 min.		30 min.		30 min.	2 hrs.	468
2	Walking		30 min.	30 min.	30 min.		30 min.	30 min.	2 hrs. 30 min.	585
3	Walk/jog		35 min.	35 min.		35 min.		35 min.	2 hrs. 20 min.	882
4										
5										
6										
7										
8										
9										
10										
11										

CRE Progress Chart

Week	Activities	Mon.	Tues.	Wed.	Thur.	Fri.	Sat.	Sun.	Weekly distance or time	Weekly calorie cost

Daily distance or time

PROFILE 13-3

Don't expect progress to be even and regular. On some days you'll feel good and your progress will be outstanding. But on other days, you'll barely be able to perform. These fluctuations are quite common—don't be concerned.

Don't rush yourself. Proceed slowly and increase your work load gradually. Your program is not for a week or a month, but for a lifetime. With a long way to go, there's no need for overzealousness, which can result in injury or enough discomfort to discourage your continued participation.

Keep in mind why you are exercising. Review your goals. If you hope to look trimmer, try to visualize what that would be like, and keep that picture in mind as an incentive to keep you going.

CONCLUDING STATEMENT

A lifestyle that strives for physical fitness contains many challenges, but the benefits are many—both in satisfactions and in pleasures. The primary challenge is related to the unfortunate fact that once developed, physical fitness is a temporary state. To retain it requires ongoing physical activity throughout life. During your college years, the facilities and environment are supportive—and you'll find many willing training partners. As you move into your professional life, your opportunities will depend on your own initiative. If you allow yourself to, you will succumb to the many distractions that are sure to plague you.

The satisfactions and pleasures of regular physical activity are self-sustaining though. And as you grow older, your energy level and capacity for enjoying recreational pursuits will remain high, and you will feel and look good. As a result, your daily physical activities will be a bright spot in your day. Be assured that your fitness lifestyle will permeate your family life too. Your spouse and children will become part of it as well, and you will feel further rewarded as those you love share your priority of physical activity as a mainstay of daily life.

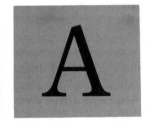

Desirable Weights for Men and Women

The tables list weights in pounds for men and women, age 25 to 59, in indoor clothing. Weights are according to height, including one-inch heels, with five pounds of clothing for men and three pounds of clothing for women. Use Profile 1-4 in Chapter 1 to help you decide whether your build is small, medium, or large.

Men

Height		Small Frame	Medium Frame	Large Frame
Feet	Inches			
5	2	128–134	131–141	138–150
5	3	130–136	133–143	140–153
5	4	132–138	135–145	142–156
5	5	134–140	137–148	144–160
5	6	136–142	139–151	146–164
5	7	138–145	142–154	149–168
5	8	140–148	145–157	152–172
5	9	142–151	148–160	155–176
5	10	144–154	151–163	158–180
5	11	146–157	154–166	161–184
6	0	149–160	157–170	164–188
6	1	152–164	160–174	168–192
6	2	155–168	164–178	172–197
6	3	158–172	167–182	176–202
6	4	162–176	171–187	181–207

SOURCE: Metropolitan Life Insurance Company.

Women

Height		Small Frame	Medium Frame	Large Frame
Feet	Inches			
4	10	102–111	109–121	118–131
4	11	103–113	111–123	120–134
5	0	104–115	113–126	122–137
5	1	106–118	115–129	125–140
5	2	108–121	118–132	128–143
5	3	111–124	121–135	131–147
5	4	114–127	124–138	134–151
5	5	117–130	127–141	137–155
5	6	120–133	130–144	140–159
5	7	123–136	133–147	143–163
5	8	126–139	136–150	146–167
5	9	129–142	139–153	149–170
5	10	132–145	142–156	152–173
5	11	135–148	145–159	155–176
6	0	138–151	148–162	158–179

SOURCE: Metropolitan Life Insurance Company.

B Sports and Activities

If you're a novice at exercise, model programs are a perfect way to get you started on improving your level of fitness. They benefit one or more of the five fitness components and can help you make progress toward achieving your fitness goals. For more experienced exercisers, however, and for those who have done the model programs and now want to supplement the routine with other less-structured forms of exercise, this chapter presents an overview of some sports and activities to choose from.

Table 1 is a comprehensive list of sports and activities. They are classified on the basis of their potential for developing each of the five fitness components. These classifications are guidelines: Certain activities may be more (or less) valuable because of differing skills, personal styles of play, and the stamina one has to keep at a sport or activity longer than usual. Also noted in the table are the skill levels required to obtain fitness benefits from the activity, the fitness prerequisite needed for participation, and how the activity is paced.

This appendix also contains brief discussions of sports and activities, including for most a chart summarizing the activity's potential for achieving each of the five fitness components and, where appropriate, the parts of the body affected (the parts most affected are listed first). Also shown in the charts for activities that provide CRE and body composition benefits is an estimate of the number of calories you burn per pound per minute.

In Table 1, the classifications of low (L), moderate (M), and high (H) for the five components of physical fitness are based on the ability of a sport or activity to develop that component.

Each sport or activity is classified for its potential value in promoting cardio-respiratory endurance (CRE). Those classified as high in CRE are the kind that can maintain the heart rate in the exercise benefit zone for at least fifteen minutes. If the activity is self-paced as well, it would be an excellent foundation for a CRE program.

TABLE 1   Summary of Sports and Activities

This table lists the sports and activities included in Chapter 7 and in this appendix, classifying them as high (H), moderate (M), or low (L) in terms of their ability to develop each of the five components of physical fitness. The skill level needed to obtain fitness benefits is noted: Low (L) means little or no skill is required to obtain fitness benefits; moderate (M) means average skill is needed to obtain fitness benefits; and high (H) means much skill is required to obtain fitness benefits. The fitness prerequisite—conditioning needs of a beginner—is also noted: Low (L) means no fitness prerequisite is required; moderate (M) means some preconditioning is required; and high (H) means substantial fitness is required. In the last column, each sport and activity is rated in terms of how it's paced: 1 means it's self-paced; 2 means it's a combination of self and others; and 3 means it's paced by someone other than yourself.

This appendix contains more information (including calorie costs) about the activities in this table. It also contains a listing for the broad category "gymnastics."

Sports and activities	Components					Skill level	Fitness prereq- uisite	How paced
	CRE	BC	MS*	ME*	F*			
Aerobic dance	H	H	M	H	H	L	L	3
Archery	L	L	L	L	L	L	L	1

258

TABLE 1   (*continued*)

Sports and activities	Components					Skill level	Fitness prerequisite	How paced
	CRE	BC	MS*	ME*	F*			
Backpacking	H	H	M	H	M	L	M	1
Badminton (skilled, singles)	H	H	M	M	M	M	M	2
Ballet	M	M	M	H	H	M	L	3
Ballroom dancing	M	M	L	M	L	M	L	3
Baseball (pitcher and catcher)	M	M	M	H	M	H	M	2
Basketball	H	H	M	H	M	M	M	2
Bicycling	H	H	M	H	M	M	L	1
Bowling	L	L	L	L	L	L	L	1
Calisthenic circuit training	H	H	M	H	M	L	L	1
Canoeing and kayaking	M	M	M	H	M	M	M	1
Cheerleading	M	M	M	M	M	M	L	3
Cross-country skiing	H	H	M	H	M	M	M	1
Fencing	M	M	M	H	H	M	L	2
Field hockey	H	H	M	H	M	M	M	2
Folk and square dancing	M	M	L	M	L	L	L	3
Football/touch	M	M	M	M	M	M	M	2
Frisbee/ultimate	H	H	M	H	M	M	M	2
Golf (riding cart)	L	L	L	L	M	L	L	1
Handball (skilled, singles)	H	H	M	H	M	M	M	2
Hiking	H	H	M	H	L	L	M	1
Hockey/ice and roller	H	H	M	H	M	M	M	2
Horseback riding	M	M	M	M	L	M	M	1
Interval circuit training	H	H	H	H	M	L	L	1
Jogging and running	H	H	M	H	L	L	L	1
Judo	M	M	H	H	M	M	L	2
Karate	H	H	M	H	H	L	M	2
Lacrosse	H	H	M	H	M	H	M	2

(continued)

TABLE 1   (*continued*)

Sports and activities	Components					Skill level	Fitness prereq- uisite	How paced
	CRE	BC	MS*	ME*	F*			
Modern dance (moving combinations)	M	M	M	H	H	L	L	3
Orienteering	H	H	M	H	L	L	M	1
Outdoor fitness trails	H	H	M	H	M	L	L	1
Popular dancing	M	M	L	M	M	M	L	3
Racquetball (skilled, singles)	H	H	M	M	M	M	M	2
Rock climbing	M	M	H	H	H	H	M	1
Rope skipping	H	H	M	H	L	M	M	1
Rowing	H	H	H	H	H	L	L	1
Rugby	H	H	M	H	M	M	M	2
Sailing	L	L	L	M	L	M	L	1
Skating/ice and roller	M	M	M	H	M	H	M	1
Skiing/Alpine	M	M	H	H	M	H	M	1
Soccer	H	H	M	H	M	M	M	2
Squash (skilled, singles)	H	H	M	M	M	M	M	2
Surfing	M	M	M	M	M	H	M	2
Swimming	H	H	M	H	M	M	L	1
Synchronized swimming	M	M	M	H	H	H	M	3
Table tennis	M	M	L	M	M	M	L	2
Tennis (skilled, singles)	H	H	M	M	M	M	M	2
Volleyball	M	M	L	M	M	M	M	2
Walking	H	H	L	M	L	L	L	1
Water polo	H	H	M	H	M	H	M	2
Waterskiing	M	M	M	H	M	H	M	2
Weight training	L	M	H	H	H	L	L	1
Wrestling	H	H	H	H	H	H	H	2
Yoga	L	L	L	M	H	H	L	1

*Ratings are for the muscle groups involved.

An activity classified as high in CRE but paced by others—either because of competition or an exercise leader—can also maintain the heart rate in the EBZ for periods of time. But because the pacing is not individualized, the heart rate could be driven above (or drop below) the EBZ for some participants. Such a sport or activity, while useful for developing CRE, should not replace a self-paced, high-CRE sport or activity as the mainstay of a fitness program.

At the other extreme, a sport or activity classified as low in CRE is one that is either anaerobic or of such low intensity that it cannot generally raise the heart rate into the EBZ. For a low-intensity sport or activity to raise the heart rate into the EBZ and thus accrue CRE benefits would require more than an hour's continuous active participation.

A sport or activity is classified as moderate, whether it's self-paced or competitively paced, because although heart rate can be brought into the EBZ, it's difficult to maintain it there for at least fifteen minutes. However, a moderate CRE activity—with its alternating periods in and out of the EBZ—can be a form of interval training, as long as the periods when the heart rate is in the EBZ last for at least two minutes at a time.

Body composition (BC), particularly reduction in body fat, is best influenced by sports or activities that are classified high in CRE. However, sport or activities classified high, or even moderate, for developing muscular endurance also help to improve body composition.

For someone interested in developing *muscular strength* (MS) and *muscular endurance* (ME), weight training is the ideal activity. It's classified high for both fitness components. A weight trainer can control the activity to a high degree and realize the potential for progressive overload by using the exact amount of weight needed to perform the repetitions required to achieve either or both muscular strength or muscular endurance. (See weight training model program in Chapter 7.)

If weight training is not feasible, there are other activities classified as high for development of muscular strength or muscular endurance. See, for example, the interval circuit training model program and calisthenic circuit training model program in Chapter 7, and isotonics, isometrics, and isokinetics in Chapter 5.

Yoga is an example of an activity high in *flexibility* (F). It puts all muscle groups and joints through a full range of movement and enables you to provide progressive overload easily and comfortably. Other activities high in flexibility include modern dance and gymnastics.

This appendix contains additional information about selected sports and activities listed in Table 1. For some sports, we show only the chart portion, classifying the activity as high (H), moderate (M), or low (L) in terms of its ability to develop each of the five components of physical fitness—cardiorespiratory endurance (CRE), body composition (BC), muscular strength (MS), muscular endurance (ME), and flexibility (F). Also given are the body parts affected and calorie information (where relevant). For many sports and activities, the chart is followed by a brief discussion of the exercise.

If the sport or activity you choose is designed to improve CRE and body composition, it would be helpful to keep track of the calories you burn. To do so, use the "Estimating calorie cost" section of the chart to get an approximate total. On many of the charts, you get a choice of calorie figures—for moderate or for vigorous exercise, say. Use whichever is more appropriate to calculate the calories burned. For example, if the chart shows that a sport or activity burns .039 calorie (for moderate exercise) per minute per pound and you weigh 140 pounds and you exercise for thirty minutes, the formula is: .039 × 140 × 30 = 164 calories burned.

Do not be misled by the seeming precision of the calorie estimates. In many cases, they represent a "best guess," based on available research supplemented by our experience and that of other authorities.

Aerobic Dance

Action	CRE	BC	MS	ME	F	Body parts affected
Moderate to vigorous	H	H	M	H	H	Legs, trunk

Estimating calorie cost

Moderate:	**.046** × your weight × total minutes in action = approximate calories burned
Vigorous:	**.062** × your weight × total minutes in action = approximate calories burned

---

Aerobic dance is a form of exercise that consists of thirty to sixty consecutive minutes of rhythmic running, hopping, skipping, jumping, sliding, stretching, and bending. It's performed to music and in response to directions called by an instructor in the manner of a square dance caller.

Classes are usually structured so that slow warm-up and stretching routines begin the session, followed by energetic and strenuous routines, and ending with slow cool-down routines. In a typical aerobic dance class, participants work at varying intensities with periodic breaks for checking the pulse. A person with low CRE can walk through some routines or do fewer repetitions while gradually building up the skill required to execute the steps and the CRE to do them at jogging or running intensities.

Aerobic dance can provide a high level of conditioning for most fitness components. It can affect the entire body, including the cardiorespiratory system. It can be the foundation of your fitness program or provide supplemental or substitute workouts in a regimen consisting of several activities. Once you learn the routines, you can practice them at home to the music of a radio, tapes, a record player, or a videotape.

A variation on aerobic dance is Jazzercise—exercises and dance steps combined into a series of dance sequences. You can do this at home, too, once you learn the basic exercises and dance steps.

Archery

	CRE	BC	MS	ME	F	Body parts affected
	L	L	L	L	L	Arms, shoulders

Backpacking (*see also* Hiking)

Action	CRE	BC	MS	ME	F	Body parts affected
With 40-lb. pack	H	H	H	H	M	Hips, thighs, lower legs, shoulders, abdominals

Estimating calorie cost

3 mph, level terrain:	$.032 \times$ your weight $\times$ total minutes in action = approximate calories burned
3.5 mph, 5° grade:	$.052 \times$ your weight $\times$ total minutes in action = approximate calories burned
3.5 mph, 15° grade:	$.078 \times$ your weight $\times$ total minutes in action = approximate calories burned
1.5 mph, 36° grade:	$.103 \times$ your weight $\times$ total minutes in action = approximate calories burned

Backpackers go hiking for more than one day at a time, carrying supplies and equipment for overnight camping in packs that may weigh twenty-five pounds or more. Like any sort of hiking, backpacking is a way to improve CRE, body composition, and muscular strength and endurance. Flexibility of the hips, knees, and ankles is an extra benefit when you hike in mountainous areas.

Beginners can benefit from a course in backpacking, either from a backpackers' club or at a local college or other institution. And plan on going out with experienced backpackers for several hikes. Try to go on a trip with no less than four people. If someone is injured, one person can remain with the injured person, while the other two seek help.

Look through some catalogs and visit stores that carry outdoor equipment before you begin to buy the equipment you need. Don't wear new boots until they're broken in to the point that they are comfortable to wear for long stretches of time. When backpacking, be sure to drink plenty of water to avoid dehydration. And, of course, give family or friends your planned trip route and schedule.

The weight of the backpack makes some preconditioning a good idea. To prepare yourself for your first hike, begin a walking or jogging model program—and give up elevators for several weeks. Neck, shoulder, and abdominal exercises will also help.

Badminton

Action	CRE	BC	MS	ME	F	Body parts affected
Skilled, singles	H	H	M	M	M	Legs
Beginner, singles; all doubles	M	M	L	L	M	Legs

Estimating calorie cost

Beginner:	$.032 \times$ your weight $\times$ total minutes in action = approximate calories burned
Skilled, doubles:	$.042 \times$ your weight $\times$ total minutes in action = approximate calories burned
Skilled, singles:	$.071 \times$ your weight $\times$ total minutes in action = approximate calories burned

Ballet

Action	CRE	BC	MS	ME	F	Body parts affected
Barre	L	M	M	H	H	Legs, hips, trunk, arms
Floor combinations	M	M	M	H	H	Legs, hips, trunk, arms

Estimating calorie cost

Floor combinations:	**.058** × your weight × total minutes in action = approximate calories burned

Ballroom Dancing

Action	CRE	BC	MS	ME	F	Body parts affected
Moderate to vigorous	M	M	L	M	L	Legs, hips

Estimating calorie cost

Moderate:	**.034** × your weight × total minutes in action = approximate calories burned
Vigorous:	**.049** × your weight × total minutes in action = approximate calories burned

Baseball and Softball

Action	CRE	BC	MS	ME	F	Body parts affected
Pitcher and catcher	M	M	M	H	M	Arms, shoulders, legs
Other players	L	L	M	M	L	Arms, shoulders, legs

Estimating calorie cost

Pitcher and catcher:	**.039** × your weight × total minutes in action = approximate calories burned

Basketball (*see also* Team Sports)

Action	CRE	BC	MS	ME	F	Body parts affected
Moderate to vigorous, half court or full court	H	H	M	H	M	Arms, hips, quadriceps, hamstrings, lower legs

Estimating calorie cost

Moderate, half court:	**.045** × your weight × total minutes in action = approximate calories burned
Moderate, full court:	**.052** × your weight × total minutes in action = approximate calories burned
Vigorous, half court:	**.071** × your weight × total minutes in action = approximate calories burned
Vigorous, full court:	**.097** × your weight × total minutes in action = approximate calories burned

Bicycling (*see also* Bicycling Program in Chapter 7)

Action	CRE	BC	MS	ME	F	Body parts affected
10 to 13 mph	H	H	M	H	M	Legs, hips

Estimating calorie cost

10 mph:	.049 × your weight × total minutes in action = approximate calories burned
13 mph:	.071 × your weight × total minutes in action = approximate calories burned

Bowling

	CRE	BC	MS	ME	F	Body parts affected
	L	L	L	L	L	Bowling arm, wrist, shoulders

Calisthenic Circuit Training (*see also* Calisthenic Circuit Training Program in Chapter 7)

Action	CRE	BC	MS	ME	F	Body parts affected
3 sets or 20 min.	M	H	M	H	M	Full body

Estimating calorie cost

3 sets or 20 min.:	.06 × your weight × total minutes in action = approximate calories burned

Canoeing and Kayaking

Action	CRE	BC	MS	ME	F	Body parts affected
Flat water, 2.5 to 4 mph	M	M	M	H	M	Arms, chest, shoulders

Estimating calorie cost

Flat water, 4 mph:*	.045 × your weight × total minutes in action = approximate calories burned

*Much higher for competitive white-water canoeing.

Canoeing differs from kayaking in the construction of the craft, the type of paddles, and how the paddles are used. The typical North American canoe is an open, rounded, hollow craft in which you kneel and paddle with a single blade. The kayak is usually smaller, lighter, and narrower, and you sit while paddling alternately with the two blades of the paddle.

The fitness level you need to use a canoe or kayak and the fitness benefits you get can vary widely. Leisurely lake paddling requires some upper-body strength and endurance. If, however, you paddle a canoe or kayak at a pace of 4 miles per hour for thirty minutes or more, you will probably find that your heart rate is in the EBZ and that significant CRE benefits can accrue. Extended outings on the water, particularly when they involve negotiating turbulent waters, or extensive training for competition requires not only high levels of fitness but considerable skill as well.

Cheerleading

Action	CRE	BC	MS	ME	F	Body parts affected
Moderate to vigorous	M	M	M	M	M	Full body

Estimating calorie cost

Moderate:	$.033$ × your weight × total minutes in action = approximate calories burned
Vigorous:	$.049$ × your weight × total minutes in action = approximate calories burned

Cross-Country Skiing

Action	CRE	BC	MS	ME	F	Body parts affected
3 to 8 mph	H	H	M	H	M	Full body

Estimating calorie cost

3 mph:	$.049$ × your weight × total minutes in action = approximate calories burned
8 mph:	$.104$ × your weight × total minutes in action = approximate calories burned

Competitive cross-country skiing is one of the most arduous athletic activities known. Some of the highest oxygen consumption levels have abeen recorded among cross-country skiers. Practiced on a regular basis, this activity has great potential for enhancing CRE and muscular endurance as well as body composition and muscular strength. Flexibility may be increased in some joints. But in general, stretching exercises are advisable both as a warm-up activity and to balance the skiing program. Cross-country skiing is most enjoyable if you are already in good shape and know how to ski. However, since it is self-paced, it can produce a training effect as long as you ski on a regular basis and gradually increase the duration, intensity, and frequency of your outings.

You can do this form of skiing wherever there is snow. Golf courses, woods, fields, snowmobile trails, and parks are all excellent terrains that require no ski lifts or fees. For your first outing, it's best to go with an experienced skier. If you begin at a pace that is comfortable for you, after an hour or two you will find that you can move along easily. By the end of the day, you should have developed at least a modicum of skill in cross-country skiing. You increase intensity with pace and by climbing hills. Brief downhill runs serve as pleasant relief intervals.

Fencing

Action	CRE	BC	MS	ME	F	Body parts affected
Moderate to vigorous	M	M	M	H	H	Fencing wrist, arm, shoulders, legs, hips

Estimating calorie cost

Moderate, drill:	**.032** × your weight × total minutes in action = approximate calories burned
Vigorous, match:	**.078** × your weight × total minutes in action = approximate calories burned

Fencing, whether with foil, épée, or saber, requires and develops muscular endurance and flexibility of the wrists, arms, and legs. It may also call for CRE if competition includes periods of intense offensive and defensive activity. These highly active bouts usually alternate with less active periods of sparring and brief intervals of rest. If continued for extended sessions, such interval training can, of course, result in CRE benefits.

Field Hockey (*see also* Team Sports)

Action	CRE	BC	MS	ME	F	Body parts affected
Moderate to vigorous	H	H	M	H	M	Legs, arms, trunk

Estimating calorie cost

Moderate:	**.052** × your weight × total minutes in action = approximate calories burned
Vigorous:	**.078** × your weight × total minutes in action = approximate calories burned

Folk and Square Dancing

Action	CRE	BC	MS	ME	F	Body parts affected
Moderate to vigorous	M	M	L	M	L	Legs, hips

Estimating calorie cost

Moderate:	**.039** × your weight × total minutes in action = approximate calories burned
Vigorous:	**.049** × your weight × total minutes in action = approximate calories burned

Football/Touch (*see also* Team Sports)

Action	CRE	BC	MS	ME	F	Body parts affected
Moderate to vigorous	M	M	M	M	M	Legs, trunk

Estimating calorie cost

Moderate:	**.049** × your weight × total minutes in action = approximate calories burned
Vigorous:	**.078** × your weight × total minutes in action = approximate calories burned

Frisbee/Ultimate (*see also* Team Sports)

Action	CRE	BC	MS	ME	F	Body parts affected
Moderate to vigorous, team	H	H	M	H	M	Legs, arms

Estimating calorie cost

Moderate, team:	**.049** × your weight × total minutes in action = approximate calories burned
Vigorous, team:	**.078** × your weight × total minutes in action = approximate calories burned

Frisbee is the trade name for a saucer-shaped plastic disc that, when tossed, sails through the air. Tossing a Frisbee to and fro can lend itself to a variety of games and activities, with a wide range of potential fitness benefits. Leisurely tossing of a Frisbee yields relatively low fitness benefits. Games such as "Ultimate Frisbee," however, use the disc actively, in the manner of basketball, field hockey, soccer, or team handball, and such sports can yield high CRE benefits. The bending and stretching required in running and jumping for a Frisbee help to promote flexibility as well.

Golf

Action	CRE	BC	MS	ME	F	Body parts affected
Riding cart	L	L	L	L	M	Legs, arms, shoulders, neck, trunk
Twosome pulling clubs, or foursome carrying clubs	L	L	M	M	M	Legs, arms, shoulders, neck, trunk
Twosome carrying clubs	M	M	M	M	M	Legs, arms, shoulders, neck, trunk

Gymnastics—Balance Beam, High Bar, Parallel Bars, Side Horse, Trampoline, Tumbling

Action	CRE	BC	MS	ME	F	Body parts affected
Moderate to vigorous	L	M	H	H	H	All

Because gymnastics requires the use of the entire body in twisting, turning, leaping, pushing, and pulling movements, it is an excellent way to improve and maintain muscular fitness.

Women's gymnastics puts greater emphasis on flexibility, while men's gymnastics puts greater emphasis on strength. Training is arduous, with the gymnast constantly working against his or her body weight. There is outstanding development of muscular strength, muscular endurance, and flexibility. And when the gymnast works continuously at a relatively high intensity for one or two hours, there are also CRE benefits.

Handball

Action	CRE	BC	MS	ME	F	Body parts affected
Skilled, singles	H	H	M	H	M	Arms, shoulders, legs
Beginner, singles; all doubles	M	M	M	M	M	Arms, shoulders, legs

Estimating calorie cost

Beginner, singles; all doubles:	.049 × your weight × total minutes in action = approximate calories burned
Skilled, singles:	.078 × your weight × total minutes in action = approximate calories burned

Inexpensive, widely available, and easy to master, handball is a popular sport. It can be played indoors or out, as singles or doubles, and with one, three, or four walls. When played at high intensity by skilled players, handball is a good way to achieve and maintain CRE and muscular endurance. Played long enough and frequently enough, it can affect body composition and be useful in weight control.

Hiking (*see also* Backpacking, Orienteering)

Action	CRE	BC	MS	ME	F	Body parts affected
2 mph with a 10-lb. pack, 10° to 20° grade	H	H	M	H	L	Hips, thighs, lower legs, shoulders, abdominals

Estimating calorie cost

2 mph, 10° grade:	.051 × your weight × total minutes in action = approximate calories burned
2 mph, 20° grade:	.073 × your weight × total minutes in action = approximate calories burned

Hiking is walking with a view. It generally means taking a day-long excursion, out and back, with a little food, drink, and emergency gear carried in a light pack. The activity is self-paced, and only minimum fitness is required to begin. The fitness benefits of hiking are similar to those of walking. You can increase distance, difficulty of terrain, and pace as fitness improves. It is wise to obtain information about trails and equipment needs beforehand and to leave your itinerary, including time schedule, with your family or friends.

Hockey/Ice and Roller (*see also* Team Sports)

Action	CRE	BC	MS	ME	F	Body parts affected
Moderate to vigorous	H	H	M	H	M	Legs, arms

Estimating calorie cost

Moderate:	.052 × your weight × total minutes in action = approximate calories burned
Vigorous:	.078 × your weight × total minutes in action = approximate calories burned

Horseback Riding

Action	CRE	BC	MS	ME	F	Body parts affected
Trot to gallop	M	M	M	M	L	Legs, trunk

Estimating calorie cost

Trot:	.052 × your weight × total minutes in action = approximate calories burned
Gallop:	.065 × your weight × total minutes in action = approximate calories burned

Interval Circuit Training (*see also* Interval Circuit Training Program in Chapter 7)

Action	CRE	BC	MS	ME	F	Body parts affected
3 sets or 20 min.	H	H	H	H	M	Full body

Estimating calorie cost

3 sets or 20 min.:	.062 × your weight × total minutes in action = approximate calories burned

Jogging and Running (*see also* Walking/Jogging/Running Model Programs in Chapter 7)

Action	CRE	BC	MS	ME	F	Body parts affected
Jog, 5 to 7 mph; run, 8 to 10 mph	H	H	M	H	L	Legs, hips

Estimating calorie cost

Slow jog, 5 mph:	.06 × your weight × total minutes in action = approximate calories burned
Fast jog, 7 mph:	.092 × your weight × total minutes in action = approximate calories burned
Slow run, 8 mph:	.104 × your weight × total minutes in action = approximate calories burned
Fast run, 10 mph:	.129 × your weight × total minutes in action = approximate calories burned

Judo

Action	CRE	BC	MS	ME	F	Body parts affected
Moderate to vigorous	M	M	H	H	M	Full body

Estimating calorie cost

Moderate:	**.049** × your weight × total minutes in action = approximate calories burned
Vigorous:	**.09** × your weight × total minutes in action = approximate calories burned

Karate

Action	CRE	BC	MS	ME	F	Body parts affected
Moderate to vigorous	H	H	M	H	H	Full body

Estimating calorie cost

Moderate:	**.049** × your weight × total minutes in action = approximate calories burned
Vigorous:	**.09** × your weight × total minutes in action = approximate calories burned

Lacrosse (*see also* Team Sports)

Action	CRE	BC	MS	ME	F	Body parts affected
Moderate to vigorous	H	H	M	H	M	Legs, arms

Estimating calorie cost

Moderate:	**.052** × your weight × total minutes in action = approximate calories burned
Vigorous:	**.078** × your weight × total minutes in action = approximate calories burned

Modern Dance

Action	CRE	BC	MS	ME	F	Body parts affected
Floor warm-ups	L	M	L	H	H	Legs, hips, trunk, arms
Moving combinations	M	M	M	H	H	Legs, hips, trunk, arms

Estimating calorie cost

Moving combinations:	**.058** × your weight × total minutes in action = approximate calories burned

Orienteering (*see also* Hiking)

Action	CRE	BC	MS	ME	F	Body parts affected
Moderate to vigorous	H	H	M	H	L	Legs

Estimating calorie cost

Moderate:	.049 × your weight × total minutes in action = approximate calories burned
Vigorous:	.078 × your weight × total minutes in action = approximate calories burned

In competitive orienteering, the object is to progress on foot over unfamiliar terrain (using only a detailed topographical map and a compass), make your way past a series of specified stations, and arrive first at the finish line. Contests are held over all types of terrain, and they last for well over an hour. Participants need speed and endurance as they sprint, jog, climb, run, and walk through the course. Although the sport emphasizes problem-solving rather than athletic ability, high levels of CRE can help considerably. Train for this activity by hiking and jogging.

Outdoor Fitness Trails *

Action	CRE	BC	MS	ME	F	Body parts affected
2.5-mile course	H	H	M	H	M	Full body

Estimating calorie cost

2.5-mile course:	.06 × your weight × total minutes in action = approximate calories burned

*Parcourse is one brand.

The outdoor fitness trail attempts to combine jogging (or walking) trails with a circuit of exercise stations. The activity originated in Switzerland in the late 1960s and is referred to as *parcours,* derived from a French term meaning "course" or "circuit." Fitness trails are receiving increased attention in the United States.

The *parcours* might be described as a "fitness playground" because of the jungle-gym nature of some of the exercise stations. Stations may number as many as twenty and vary in type as well as materials used. The total distance of the course also varies, depending on how far apart the stations are. The course may extend from about ¾ of a mile up to 2½ miles. Participants do sit-ups, pull-ups, or other exercises at each of the stations, then walk, jog, or run along the trail or path to the next station.

A typical course begins with a detailed map of the course and a description of how it is to be used. Directional signs guide you toward the stations. Each station has a sign that illustrates and explains how the exercise is to be performed and the number of repetitions of the exercise.

The outdoor fitness trail can serve as a good all-around fitness program for some people. The fact that it is outdoors offers a varied and attractive challenge that may be appealing. However, the potential fitness benefits of a particular trail will depend on whether the exercise stations are designed to develop muscular strength, endurance, and flexibility of all major muscle groups and whether the exerciser participates at an intensity high enough to maintain the heart rate within the EBZ for at least fifteen minutes and preferably longer.

Popular Dancing

Action	CRE	BC	MS	ME	F	Body parts affected
Vigorous	M	M	L	M	M	Legs, hips

Estimating calorie cost

Vigorous:	.049 × your weight × total minutes in action = approximate calories burned

Racquetball

Action	CRE	BC	MS	ME	F	Body parts affected
Skilled, singles	H	H	M	M	M	One side of body, trunk, legs
Beginner, singles; all doubles	M	M	M	M	M	One side of body, trunk, legs

Estimating calorie cost

Beginner, singles; all doubles:	.049 × your weight × total minutes in action = approximate calories burned
Skilled, singles:	.078 × your weight × total minutes in action = approximate calories burned

One of the fastest growing sports in the United States, racquetball is played on a court similar to the one used in four-wall handball. Racquetball is played with a short-handled racket, strung like a tennis racket. A principal attraction of racquetball for many is its potential for developing CRE without requiring more than modest skill.

Rock Climbing

Action	CRE	BC	MS	ME	F	Body parts affected
Moderate to vigorous	M	M	H	H	H	Full body

Estimating calorie cost

Moderate to vigorous:	.033 × your weight × total minutes in action = approximate calories burned

Rock climbing involves ascending and descending steep cliffs or rock faces by means of hand and foot holds.

The activity requires—and will develop—muscular strength, muscular endurance, and flexibility. Pulling yourself up and stretching to reach the hand and foot holds contribute to these fitness components. *Belaying* (holding the safety ropes for your partner) and *rappelling* (rapid descent using a rope) require rope-handling skills and contribute to muscular strength and endurance. But rock climbing contributes moderately to CRE because the pace is generally slow, and there are usually frequent rest periods.

Rope Skipping (*see also* Rope Skipping Program in Chapter 7)

Action	CRE	BC	MS	ME	F	Body parts affected
70 to 100 turns per min.	H	H	M	H	L	Legs, forearms

Estimating calorie cost

70 turns per min.:	**.071** × your weight × total minutes in action = approximate calories burned
80 turns per min.:	**.079** × your weight × total minutes in action = approximate calories burned
90 turns per min.:	**.087** × your weight × total minutes in action = approximate calories burned
100 turns per min.:	**.095** × your weight × total minutes in action = approximate calories burned

Rowing

Action	CRE	BC	MS	ME	F	Body parts affected
Moderate to vigorous	H	H	H	H	H	Full body

Estimating calorie cost

Moderate:	**.032** × your weight × total minutes in action = approximate calories burned
Vigorous:	**.097** × your weight × total minutes in action = approximate calories burned

Competitive rowing—including *sweeps,* in which each crew member uses only one oar, and *sculls,* in which each person uses two—activates many major muscle groups. It is an excellent way to develop all the fitness components. (In a rowboat without a sliding seat, however, one gets little activity in the thigh muscles, thus limiting the CRE benefits derived from the sport.)

Practice sessions often involve one or two hours of high-intensity exercise, burning lots of calories and achieving CRE and body composition goals. Strenuous rowing, whether in an actual boat or a stationary rowing machine, also provides high levels of muscular strength, muscular endurance, and flexibility.

Recreational rowing in a traditional flat-bottomed rowboat can also be a good fitness activity if you row at adequate levels of intensity, duration, and frequency. Stationary rowing should provide similar benefits to regular rowing.

Rugby (*see also* Team Sports)

Action	CRE	BC	MS	ME	F	Body parts affected
Moderate to vigorous	H	H	M	H	M	Legs, trunk, arms, shoulders

Estimating calorie cost

Moderate:	**.052** × your weight × total minutes in action = approximate calories burned
Vigorous:	**.097** × your weight × total minutes in action = approximate calories burned

Sailing

	CRE	BC	MS	ME	F	Body parts affected
	L	L	L	M	L	Arms, shoulders, trunk

Skating/Ice and Roller

Action	CRE	BC	MS	ME	F	Body parts affected
Beginner to vigorous	M	M	M	H	M	Legs, hips

Estimating calorie cost

Beginner:	$.032 \times$ your weight $\times$ total minutes in action = approximate calories burned
Moderate:	$.049 \times$ your weight $\times$ total minutes in action = approximate calories burned
Vigorous:	$.065 \times$ your weight $\times$ total minutes in action = approximate calories burned

Most variants of ice and roller skating require rhythmic large-muscle movements capable of developing CRE, improving body composition, and burning a great many calories over a long duration. To do this, of course, you must skate at high intensity for fifteen minutes or more at least three times a week.

It may take some time to develop sufficient skill to use skating as a fitness exercise, but once you can skate well enough to enjoy the recreational and social aspects, you should be able to skate hard and fast enough to get your heart rate into the EBZ and achieve a CRE training effect. In addition to CRE, skating can improve flexibility, muscular endurance, and muscular strength, especially in the legs and hips.

Skiing/Alpine

Action	CRE	BC	MS	ME	F	Body parts affected
Continuous, intermediate to expert	M	M	H	H	M	Thighs, hips

Estimating calorie cost

Continuous, intermediate:	$.039 \times$ your weight $\times$ total minutes in action = approximate calories burned
Continuous, expert:	$.078 \times$ your weight $\times$ total minutes in action = approximate calories burned

Alpine, or downhill, skiing can develop moderate-to-high levels of fitness, depending on how well you ski and how fit you are to begin with. With moderate skill, skiing can supplement your regular fitness program, particularly in developing muscular strength and endurance in the thighs and hips.

If your ski runs exceed five to ten minutes, and if you can repeat them throughout the day—using the lift ride as a rest interval—you may even achieve some CRE benefits as well. Of course, you can modify your pace and select trails of varying difficulty to get the effect of interval training. High-intensity skiing requires muscular strength and endurance as well as high CRE. Be sure to warm up and cool down adequately before and after each outing. However, because skiing for most people is only a weekend recreational activity, you will not be able to depend on it as the mainstay of a fitness program.

Soccer (*see also* Team Sports)

Action	CRE	BC	MS	ME	F	Body parts affected
Moderate to vigorous	H	H	M	H	M	Legs, trunk, neck

Estimating calorie cost

Moderate:	.052 × your weight × total minutes in action = approximate calories burned
Vigorous:	.097 × your weight × total minutes in action = approximate calories burned

Squash

Action	CRE	BC	MS	ME	F	Body parts affected
Skilled, singles	H	H	M	M	M	Arms, shoulders
Beginner, singles; all doubles	M	M	M	M	M	Arms, shoulders

Estimating calorie cost

Beginner, singles; all doubles:	.049 × your weight × total minutes in action = approximate calories burned
Skilled, singles:	.078 × your weight × total minutes in action = approximate calories burned

One of the fastest of all the racquet sports, squash (also known as squash racquets) is played on a small four-walled indoor court. Players must move fast, not only to get into position to return their opponent's shots, but also to keep out of each other's way in the limited playing area. Many people play squash because it provides an intense workout in a short space of time.

Surfing

Action	CRE	BC	MS	ME	F	Body parts affected
Including swimming	M	M	M	M	M	Legs, upper body

Estimating calorie cost

Including swimming:	.078 × your weight × total minutes in action = approximate calories burned

Riding a surfboard over waves that move in toward a beach can be a vigorous activity capable of developing all five fitness components, if you continue the activity for extended periods of time on a regular basis. The major fitness benefits are derived before the actual surfing takes place—that is, while paddling the surfboard away from the shore toward the breaking waves. Paddling out, like swimming, works the muscles of the chest, arms, and shoulders. This may put surfers into the EBZ before they even begin to mount and balance themselves on their boards. While riding the board, skilled surfers often execute maneuvers requiring considerable athletic ability and fitness. They need excellent CRE and swimming skills to keep afloat in turbulent water for fifteen to thirty minutes.

Swimming (*see also* Swimming Program in Chapter 7)

Action	CRE	BC	MS	ME	F	Body parts affected
20 to 55 yds. per min.	H	H	M	H	M	Arms, shoulders, chest

Estimating calorie cost

20 yds. per min.:	$.032 \times$ your weight $\times$ total minutes in action = approximate calories burned
55 yds. per min.:	$.088 \times$ your weight $\times$ total minutes in action = approximate calories burned

Synchronized Swimming

Action	CRE	BC	MS	ME	F	Body parts affected
Moderate to vigorous	M	M	M	H	H	Full body

Estimating calorie cost

Moderate:	$.032 \times$ your weight $\times$ total minutes in action = approximate calories burned
Vigorous:	$.052 \times$ your weight $\times$ total minutes in action = approximate calories burned

Synchronized swimming (water ballet) is a group water activity performed in choreographed patterns in time to music. This combination of art and sport requires strong, proficient swimming skills, flexibility, and moderate-to-high levels of CRE and muscular endurance. Proficiency requires long hours of practice, usually as a member of a team or club representing a school or "Y." Practice sessions last at least an hour at a time and take place on a regular basis. This form of swimming is particularly helpful in developing flexibility and can produce training effects in CRE and muscular endurance equal to those of a swimming program.

Table Tennis

Action	CRE	BC	MS	ME	F	Body parts affected
Skilled	M	M	L	M	M	One side of body, wrist, arm

Estimating calorie cost

Skilled:	.045 × your weight × total minutes in action = approximate calories burned

The United States Table Tennis Association notes that the sport of table tennis, also known as Ping-Pong, is the second most popular participation sport in the world, surpassed only by soccer. Perhaps this is so because it's a game that allows people of any sex, age, size, and strength to play.

This game is a form of tennis played on a table. It can be played for fun—a leisurely, low-intensity game—or it can be quite vigorous, depending on the skills of the players. The fitness benefits, however, can be limited by a player's inability to perform at high skill levels or by lack of stiff competition.

Team Sports (*see* Basketball, Field Hockey, Football/Touch, Frisbee/Ultimate, Hockey/Ice and Roller, Lacrosse, Rugby, Soccer)

The running and skating team sports—basketball; field, ice, and roller hockey; football; lacrosse; rugby; soccer; and ultimate Frisbee—are highly competitive team games in which each team defends its goal against running and passing attacks from the opposing team. These games all require more or less continuous movement up, down, and across a field, court, or rink. So they demand and produce moderate-to-high levels of CRE and muscular endurance in the legs. The speed and continuity of the running or skating vary from sport to sport and from time to time within any game, with short bursts of speed followed by more leisurely runs (as in basketball or soccer) or with frequent shifting of personnel (as in the two-platoon system in football). Intensity also varies with the position you play. For example, the center-halfback on a soccer team is generally more active than a fullback, who may be relatively inactive if the team's offensive unit is dominating the game.

The major fitness benefits acquired from these sports come from practice sessions. In organized teams, these usually include warm-up exercises, jogging, and weight training, as well as fast-moving drills and scrimmages. By improving your flexibility, muscular development, body composition, and CRE—both during the playing season and in the off-season—you can improve your performance, increase your protection against injury, and gain greater enjoyment on the playing field.

Tennis

Action	CRE	BC	MS	ME	F	Body parts affected
Skilled, singles	H	H	M	M	M	One side of body, playing arm, shoulder, legs
Beginner, singles; all doubles	M	M	M	M	M	One side of body, playing arm, shoulder, legs

Estimating calorie cost

Beginner:	.032 × your weight × total minutes in action = approximate calories burned
Skilled, doubles:	.049 × your weight × total minutes in action = approximate calories burned
Skilled, singles:	.071 × your weight × total minutes in action = approximate calories burned

Tennis requires good eye-hand coordination. It also demands speed and agility to get yourself into position to return the ball once your opponent has hit it to your side of the net. The intensity of play varies widely, depending on your skill and the skill of your opponent, the surface of the court, and especially on whether you are playing singles or doubles. In singles, you cover your entire side of the court, which could require a great deal of running with rapid starts and short stops. In doubles, partners take turns both serving and returning balls; they run less and hit fewer shots. You probably cannot rely on tennis to produce significant benefits in CRE or body composition, unless you are highly skilled and play frequently and for long durations. You can achieve a limited amount of muscular strength and endurance, especially in the legs and the playing arm and shoulder.

The game requires a high degree of skill; lessons are recommended to get started.

Track and Field

Track and field is a general term covering competitive walking, running, jumping, and throwing events. The walking and running events are held on a track and may range from a short sprint to a six-mile run. Running events also include hurdle racing, which requires jumping over obstacles. Jumping events include the high jump, running broad jump, triple jump, and pole vault. Throwing, jumping, and short-distance sprinting events require power. Muscular strength, then, is an important fitness component in performing these events—hence the critical role of weight training in preparation for track and field events. Muscular endurance and flexibility are also necessary. The particular muscle groups to receive special attention depend on the event. The explosive events such as the jumps and sprints require anaerobic fitness. CRE is the component most necessary for (and developed by) distance runners and walkers.

Track and field enthusiasts who are serious about their participation and adhere to any of the typical, currently accepted training regimens will usually have a high level of fitness for all components.

Volleyball

Action	CRE	BC	MS	ME	F	Body parts affected
Moderate to vigorous	M	M	L	M	M	Arms, shoulders

Estimating calorie cost

Vigorous (skilled, competitive):	.065 × your weight × total minutes in action = approximate calories burned

The fitness benefits of volleyball can range from minimal to considerable, depending on the skills of the players and the conditions under which the game is played. Most of us are familiar with beach or backyard volleyball, involving people of all ages, sexes, and skills. The games can be fun, but they are actually of little fitness value. Competitive volleyball is a different story. Played at the high school, intercollegiate, amateur, and even Olympic levels, it has grown increasingly popular in recent years. At these levels, volleyball includes vigorous leaping, spiking, blocking, and diving; and it can develop CRE as well as muscular endurance and flexibility. These fitness benefits are particularly available to members of an established team that practices regularly for one to two hours each session.

Walking (*see also* Walking/Jogging/Running Model Programs in Chapter 7)

Action	CRE	BC	MS	ME	F	Body parts affected
Slow to fast walk, 2.5 to 4.5 mph	H	H	L	H	L	Hips, legs

Estimating calorie cost

Moderate, 3.5 mph:	.029 × your weight × total minutes in action = approximate calories burned
Fast, 4.5 mph:	.048 × your weight × total minutes in action = approximate calories burned

Water Polo

Action	CRE	BC	MS	ME	F	Body parts affected
Vigorous	H	H	M	H	M	Arms, shoulders, legs

Estimating calorie cost

Vigorous:	.078 × your weight × total minutes in action = approximate calories burned

Water polo, a game like field hockey or football but played in a lake or swimming pool, is a rough contact sport. Swimmers score points by shooting a ball slightly smaller than a basketball into a net in the pool. Players must be fast and skillful swimmers with high levels of muscular endurance and CRE. They must be able to change swimming directions without losing time or momentum and with or without the ball. Training for and participation in water polo can develop all five fitness components.

Waterskiing

Action	CRE	BC	MS	ME	F	Body parts affected
Moderate to vigorous	M	M	M	H	M	Arms, thighs

Estimating calorie cost

Moderate:	.039 × your weight × total minutes in action = approximate calories burned
Vigorous:	.055 × your weight × total minutes in action = approximate calories burned

Waterskiing requires and can develop muscular endurance of the arms and thighs. Its value for CRE depends on whether the skier has adequate skill and muscular endurance to sustain fifteen minutes of continuous waterskiing. If you water-ski three or four times a week and can do intermediate and advanced skiing maneuvers, waterskiing can serve as a good fitness activity.

Weight Training (*see also* Weight Training Program in Chapter 7)

	CRE	BC	MS	ME	F	Body parts affected
	L	M	H	H	H	Full body

Wrestling

Action	CRE	BC	MS	ME	F	Body parts affected
Moderate to vigorous	H	H	H	H	H	Full body

Estimating calorie cost

Moderate:	.065 × your weight × total minutes in action = approximate calories burned
Vigorous, competitive:	.094 × your weight × total minutes in action = approximate calories burned

A demanding sport, wrestling requires a high level of conditioning in each of the fitness components. Practice sessions last at least an hour. Typically, they include a warm-up period with considerable stretching, followed by a long session of drill on the many offensive and defensive maneuvers. These are followed by sparring matches, organized by weight classification. The vigorous activity can promote muscular endurance as well as CRE. The resistance offered by opponents improves muscular strength and provides the necessary twisting and turning to develop flexibility.

Yoga

	CRE	BC	MS	ME	F	Body parts affected
	L	L	L	M	H	Full body

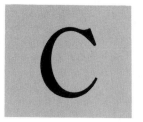

Food Exchange Plan

Lean Meat: 1 exchange = 55 calories

Beef: Baby beef, chipped beef, chuck, flank steak, tenderloin, plate ribs, plate skirt steak, round, rump, spare ribs, tripe	1 oz.
Lamb: Leg, rib, sirloin, loin, shank, shoulder	1 oz.
Pork: Leg, ham, smoked (center slices)	1 oz.
Veal: Leg, loin, rib, shank, shoulder, cutlets	1 oz.
Poultry: Chicken, turkey, Cornish hen, guinea hen, pheasant (all without skin)	1 oz.
Fish: Any fresh or frozen	1 oz.
Canned salmon, tuna, mackerel, crab, lobster	¼ cup
Clams, oysters, scallops, shrimp	5 or 1 oz.
Sardines, drained	3
Cheeses: containing less than 5% butterfat	1 oz.
Cottage cheese: dry or 2% butterfat	¼ cup
Dried beans and peas (omit 1 bread exchange)	½ cup

Medium-Fat Meat: 1 exchange = 78 calories *(Omit ½ fat exchange)*

Beef: Ground (15% fat), corned beef (canned), rib eye, round (ground commercial)	1 oz.
Pork: Loin (all cuts tenderloin), shoulder arm (picnic), shoulder blade, Boston butt, Canadian bacon, boiled ham	1 oz.
Liver, heart, kidney, sweetbreads	1 oz.
Cottage cheese: creamed	¼ cup
Cheeses: Mozzarella, ricotta, farmers, neufchatel	1 oz.
Parmesan cheese	3 T.
Egg	1
Peanut butter *(omit 2 additional fat exchanges)*	2 T.

High-Fat Meat: 1 exchange = 100 calories *(Omit 1 fat exchange)*

Beef: Brisket, corned beef (brisket), ground beef (more than 20% fat), hamburger (commercial), chuck (ground commercial), roasts (rib), steaks (club and rib)	1 oz.
Lamb: Breast	1 oz.
Pork: Spareribs, loin (back ribs), pork (ground), country style ham, deviled ham	1 oz.
Veal: Breast	1 oz.
Poultry: Capon, duck (domestic), goose	1 oz.
Cheese: Cheddar types	1 oz.
Cold cuts	4½″ × ⅛″ slice
Frankfurter	1 small

FAT EXCHANGE: 1 EXCHANGE = 45 CALORIES

Butter, margarine, mayonnaise, oil, lard, bacon fat	1 tsp.
Margarine, diet	2 tsp.
Avocado (4″ diameter)	⅛
Olives	5 small
Almonds	10 whole
Pecans	2 large, whole
Peanuts	
Spanish	20 whole
Virginia	10 whole
Walnuts and other nuts	6 small
Bacon, crisp	1 strip
Cream, light or sour	2 T.
Cream, heavy	1 T.
Cream cheese	1 T.
French or Italian dressing	1 T.
Mayonnaise	1 tsp.
Mayonnaise, imitation or diet	2 tsp.
Salad dressing, low calorie	2 tsp.

BREAD EXCHANGE (INCLUDES BREAD, CEREAL, AND STARCHY VEGETABLES): 1 EXCHANGE = 70 CALORIES

Bread: White, whole wheat, rye pumpernickel, rye, raisin	1 slice
Rolls: Bagel, English muffin, frankfurter or hamburger roll	½
Plain dinner roll	1
Tortilla, 6″	1
Pita bread (pocket bread)	½
Bread crumbs, dried	3 T.
Cereal	
Ready to serve, unsweetened variety	¾ cup
Cooked	½ cup
Popcorn (popped, no fat added)	3 cups
Cornmeal, dry	2 T.
Flour	2½ T.
Wheat Germ	¼ cup
Grits (cooked)	½ cup
Pasta (cooked): Spaghetti, noodles, macaroni, rice, barley	½ cup
Crackers	
Graham	2 squares
Matzoh, 4″ × 6″	½
Oyster	20
Ritz	5
Saltines	6
Pretzels, 3⅛″ × ⅛″	25

Legumes

Beans, baked	¼ cup
Dried beans, kidney, lima, navy, pinto, red, chick-peas, black-eyed peas, split peas	½ cup

Starchy vegetables

Corn	⅓ cup
Corn on the cob	1 small
Lima beans, mashed potatoes, winter squash	½ cup
Parsnips	¾ cup
Peas, green	¾ cup

Potato, white or sweet	1 medium
Pumpkin	¾ cup
Yams	¼ cup

Prepared foods

Biscuit or muffin, 2″ (omit 1 fat exchange)	1
Cornbread, 2″ × 2″ × 1″ (omit 1 fat exchange)	1
Potatoes, French fried, 2″ × 3½″ (omit 1 fat exchange)	8
Potato or corn chips (omit 2 fat exchanges)	15
Pancake or waffle, 5″ × ½″ (omit 1 fat exchange)	1

MILK EXCHANGE: 1 EXCHANGE = 80 CALORIES

Nonfat

Skim	1 cup
Powder, dry	⅓ cup
Evaporated, skim	½ cup
Buttermilk	1 cup
Yogurt, plain, unflavored	1 cup

Low-fat (omit 1 fat exchange)

2% fat	1 cup
Yogurt, 2% plain, unflavored	1 cup

Whole (omit 2 fat exchanges)

Whole milk	1 cup
Evaporated, whole	½ cup
Buttermilk, whole	1 cup
Yogurt, whole, plain, unflavored	1 cup

VEGETABLE EXCHANGE: 1 EXCHANGE = 25 CALORIES

Group A: ½-cup serving

Artichokes, hearts	Broccoli	Chinese pea pods
Asparagus	Brussels sprouts	Eggplant
Bean sprouts	Cabbage	Green pepper
Beets	Carrots	Greens

Kohlrabi	String beans, green or yellow	Turnips
Okra	Summer squash	Water chestnuts
Onion	Tomatoes (1 small)	Zucchini
Rutabaga	Tomato juice, vegetable juice	

Group B: Serving size—no more than amounts shown below

Cauliflower	1½ cups	Lettuce	2 cups
Celery	1 cup	Mushrooms	1 cup
Chicory	2 cups	Parsley	2 cups
Chinese cabbage	2 cups	Radishes	2 cups
Cucumbers	2 cups	Rhubarb	1 cup
Endive	1½ cups	Sauerkraut	1 cup
Escarole	1½ cups	Watercress	2 cups

Fruit Exchange: 1 exchange = 40 calories

Apple	1 small
Apple juice, apple cider	⅓ cup
Applesauce (unsweetened)	½ cup
Apricots, fresh	2 med.
Apricots, dried	4 halves
Banana	½ small
Berries	
Blackberries	½ cup
Blueberries	½ cup
Raspberries	½ cup
Strawberries	¾ cup
Cherries	10 large
Cranberries	1 cup
Dates	2
Figs, fresh or dry	1
Grapefruit	½
Grapefruit juice	½ cup
Grapes	12
Grape juice	¼ cup
Mango	½ small
Melon	
Cantaloupe	¼ medium
Honeydew	⅛ medium
Watermelon	1 cup
Nectarine	1 small
Orange	1 small
Orange juice	½ cup
Papaya	¾ cup
Peach	1 small
Pear	1 small
Pineapple	½ cup

Pineapple juice	⅓ cup
Plums	2 medium
Prunes	2 medium
Prune juice	¼ cup
Raisins	2 T.
Tangerine	1 medium

MISCELLANEOUS EXCHANGE (NO NUTRITIONAL VALUE): 1 EXCHANGE = 50 CALORIES

Hard candy (small) or caramel	1
Sugar, syrup, honey, jam, jelly, cocoa	1 level T.

FREE FOODS (NEGLIGIBLE CALORIES)

Bouillon, broth	Pickles (unsweetened)
Coffee, tea	Mustard, soy sauce, vinegar
Herbs, spices	Diet soda
Gelatin, plain and rennet tablets	Saccharin
Lemon juice, lime juice	

BONUS FOODS (LIMIT TO 2 TIMES PER WEEK):*

Frozen low-fat yogurt	6 oz.	150 cal.	Omit 1 milk + 1 fat exchange
Ice cream	½ cup	150 cal.	Omit 1 milk + 1 fat exchange
Cake/icing	¹⁄₁₂	200 cal.	Omit 1 bread + 2 fat exchanges
Angelfood cake, no icing	¹⁄₁₆	110 cal.	Omit 1 bread + 1 fat exchange
Wine, dry	6 oz.	150 cal.	Omit 1 bread + 1 misc. exchange
Wine, sweet	4 oz.	150 cal.	Omit 1 bread + 1 misc. exchange
Beer	12 oz.	150 cal.	Omit 1 bread + 1 misc. exchange
Liquor (whiskey, gin, bourbon)	1 oz.	65 cal.	Omit 1 bread exchange
Pie, 9″	¹⁄₁₂	200 cal.	Omit 1 bread + 2 fat exchanges
Cheesecake, 8″	⅙	200 cal.	Omit 1 bread + 2 fat exchanges
Pizza, 10″	¼	250 cal.	Omit 2 bread + 2 fat exchanges
Cookies	2	150 cal.	Omit 1 bread + 1 fat exchange

*These bonus foods are intended for only *occasional use*—no more than twice a week. The exchanges you are asked to omit are not exact equivalents for the bonus foods but are approximations intended to provide a fairly balanced intake.

Index